Nourishing the Body
and
Recovering Health

Praise for
Nourishing the Body
and
Recovering Health

"If you've ever considered upgrading your diet and creating a healthier you, this book is for you. It's written by a physician who has taken the time to explore the real science (as opposed to that funded by the junk food industry). She writes clearly and positively about the wonderful benefits that are waiting for you, and tells you precisely what you can do to obtain far more health, joy and personal power. Highly recommended."

—John Robbins, author *Diet For A New America, The Food Revolution*, and President of The Food Revolution Network

"Packed with inspiration and practical wisdom, it is a joyous tour-de-force for transforming one's health and life through food."

—Jonathan Balcombe, PhD, author of *Pleasurable Kingdom*

"Ana Negrón's book is an alchemical wonder. In it, Dr. Negrón combines the hard-nosed rigor of a scientist, the non-nonsense clarity of a great family doctor, the cheerful efficiency of a top-notch life coach, and the compassionate soul of a loving abuelita. Through stories, examples, exercises, recipes, and practical tips, Dr. Negrón empowers readers to recover their own health and share the gift of vibrant well-being with loved ones. Anyone who adopts this book as their guide will discover an easy and pleasant journey to an incredible destination."

—Howard Jacobson, PhD, contributing author to *Whole: Rethinking the Science of Nutrition*, and host of the Plant Yourself Podcast

"Ana M. Negrón moves from the doctor's office to the kitchen, in pursuit of preventive measures to help her patients, as well as the public. From treating diabetes to preventing heart disease, the answers to today's health crisis may be found on the dinner plate. Negrón provides clear and specific diet strategies to take charge of your health once and for all."

—Sharon Palmer, RDN, registered dietitian nutritionist, and author of *Plant-Powered for Life*

"Informative, motivating and empowering. With wisdom, practicality, and grace, Dr. Negrón slips into your kitchen and your head. Let her in and she will change your life.
—Susan Silberstein, PhD, author of *Hungry for Health* and *Hungrier for Health*

"This book serves as a ray of hope for those who are looking for a healthy way of being in a society where obesity has become pandemic. It diagnoses the condition of our society and prescribes a no nonsense and out of the ordinary approach to better health and long life. Thank you Dr. Negrón for this much needed guide for a simple and plant based diet for a healthy America."
—The Rev. Koshy Mathews, DMin, Rector, St. Peter's Episcopal Church in Phoenixville

"Dr. Ana Negrón is a teacher, coach, and motivator as she guides you on a journey to eating well and feeling new energy and health. As the 'guide by your side' she helps you to transition from your current eating habits to a nutritious approach that celebrates the untapped potential of our bodies and how we can feel. This comprehensive book is at times hard hitting against the food industry and, dear to my own heart, schools—what our children are eating in school cafeterias and what they learn or do not learn about food in the curriculum. However, it offers positive recommendations and suggestions for moving in a new direction. You can learn how to set up your own home kitchen and make the creation of healthy meals a family event. This is a very enjoyable book filled with anecdotes, menus, action plans, practical approaches, and words of encouragement for 'people in progress.' Parents, teachers, school leaders, and all of those charged with the care of our children should read this important book. Dr. Negrón knows that changing what and how we eat may not be easy, but the benefits are an investment in our children and ourselves."
—Thomas L. Tobin, EdD, former School Principal, Assistant Superintendent, and Teacher Principal of Two National Blue Ribbon Schools

"I stand in awe of Dr. Negrón's integrity, and commitment to delivering the message that food literacy and what we eat heals and sustains our lives. After decades on medicine for chronic diagnoses, my path crossed with Dr. Negrón. Twenty-one days of plant-based eating resulted in coming off my medicines, with energy restored. Dr. Negrón's book, written for those of us new to exploring food as medicine, as well as for medical professionals changing course in realizing the healing benefits of food over medicine, has become my nutrition Bible, always within arm's reach."

—Jane Heil

"I have been farming fruits and vegetables for 20 years and during that time I have seen the average Americans diet become increasingly worse. In our society instant gratification often plays a large part in the food choices we make. In this book Dr. Negrón answers the serious question of why we as a society are failing our bodies and our health through the food choices we make. By taking a look at not just how we eat but why we make the food choices we do, she is able to deconstruct our societies poor eating patterns and build a case for how we can all change our diets and in turn make ourselves better through food. It is a message that resonates to those who have too often relied on medications for ailments without realizing that health can be changed through diet in a simple and cost effective way."

—Fred de Long, Director, Willistown Conservation Trust Community Farm Program

"Ana's knowledge, insight and caring have helped relieve me of constant body pain of fifteen years duration. By choosing foods that soothe and nourish my body rather than inflame it, I've been able to resume activities, greet each day with a healthy store of energy and live a more effective Life. Ana gives detailed information on the basics and complexities of working through inflammation, releasing dependency on medications, and achieving balance through a proven approach to meeting nutritional needs. She will take you, step by step, into an experience of health you may have thought impossible."

—Sharon Wylie, collage artist

"I've worked for nearly 20 years with Dr. Negrón. Teaching family physicians about food literacy and helping patients develop healthier lifestyles, her insights, passion, focus, and intensity are all evident in this compelling book. It lays out in organized fashion some of the folly of American medicine and specific ways people can take their future health into their own hands with the food choices they make."

—Barry J. Jacobs, PsyD, Director of Behavioral Sciences, Crozer-Keystone Family Medicine Residency, author of *The Emotional Survival Guide for Caregivers*

"Dr. Negrón has written a fantastic book that I regard as a workbook for healthy eating. Anyone interested in improving his health with lifestyle change should engage this workbook. I am particularly impressed with the impact of Dr. Negrón's recipes and food photos on a transformation to better health."

—Jeffrey I. Mechanick, M.D., Endocrinologist, Immediate Past President American Association of Clinical Endocrinologists

"As a physician in family practice, Dr. Negrón became disillusioned with the standard medical model of treating multiple symptoms of bad nutrition by dispensing expensive drugs to her patients and instead established a more preventive approach, educating them about food choices based on science and physiological fact rather than ad slogans and corporate profits. This book grew out of that commitment and promises to bring her clear-eyed message to the public at large, who are still bombarded by myth-based recommendations such as low-carb diets, paleo diets, 'butter is back' and the latest apologia for 'necessary' meat and dairy consumption. It will foster a nutritional literacy in the reader allowing her or him to evaluate claims and make choices to improve bodily health rather than those of the standard American diet that so often foster the development of chronic diseases. Dr. Negrón has long been an articulate advocate for sensible plant-based eating and for an educated, fully aware populace that makes positive, informed decisions about food, and this book can only contribute to moving consumers and would-be patients further toward that goal."

—Vance Lehmkuhl, V for Veg, *Philadelphia Daily News*

"I have known Ana Negrón since she first signed up for my food literacy training in Philadelphia in 2000. The fact that she realized the importance of food in healing and wanted to bring this information to her patients demonstrates her insightful concern for her patients and devotion to the healing arts. Ana proudly conducts cooking/nutrition workshops for her patients with diet-related diseases and thereby provides them with the life skills they need to be in charge of their health as well as experiencing the joy of beautiful, health-promoting foods. Dr. Negrón is a model of all that is good in medical care.

—Antonia Demas, PhD, President, Food Studies Institute

"Dr. Negrón guides the reader to make realistic lifestyle changes by introducing the healing potential that is inherent in a plant-based diet. This book is rich with information and poignant case studies, providing inspiration to make healthy life changes."

—Veda Andrus, EdD, MSN, RN, HN-BC; Vice President, Education and Program Development; The BirchTree Center for Healthcare Transformation

"As educators, we want to empower children and teenagers to make good choices in many facets of their lives. Most of what we want them to be able do in life is the result of a healthy body and mind. Dr. Ana Negrón's book can be summarized by the quote, 'Eat well, live well.' If you are looking for a guide to better health and wellness through nourishment, this book is a curricular guide for healthy eating. It integrates the physical, earth and life sciences with food and health care.

"Our nutritional choices affect our health and our health also affects others. Dr. Negrón highlights that it's a personal responsibility to eat as nutritiously as we can. Her recommendations are supported by scientific findings and examples. You will find some of her comments amusing yet thought provoking.

"'Knowledge is Power' and Dr. Negrón shares information that will assist you in changing your regular food choices with food that is not only nutritional but also tastes good. Her research confirms that when you nourish the body, your medical costs are lower because you are healthier and you are better able to fight disease. Childhood obesity is on the rise. School Districts need to take note on the advice given by Dr. Negrón on how they can improve their school lunch program. By eating nutritiously our bodies have more energy and we are able to maintain a healthy body weight at any age.

"My colleagues and I look forward to Dr. Ana Negrón's book to enhance our instruction and practices in public schools."

—Anthony J. Sparano, Jr. MEd, Elementary Principal,
Pennsylvania's National Distinguished Principal, 2014

"In her book, Ana Negrón writes a new prescription which guides us to nourish our body and transform our health and well-being. Through health literacy and cooking with her patients, Dr. Negrón offers a new model of care that not only promotes individual health but has a ripple effect to the health of the community and healthcare as a whole. In her book, she offers a practical step by step approach which makes the process of reaching health goals achievable and even an enjoyable process. In her book, Dr. Negrón helps us to understand the positive science of food and how adopting a whole food plant based diet can help us heal and thrive. I have experienced many positive benefits in my own health from her wisdom. I am grateful to Dr. Negrón for lighting the way. This book will be my continued source of inspiration."

—Eileen Bowe, MSN, CRNP, Cardiology Nurse Practitioner

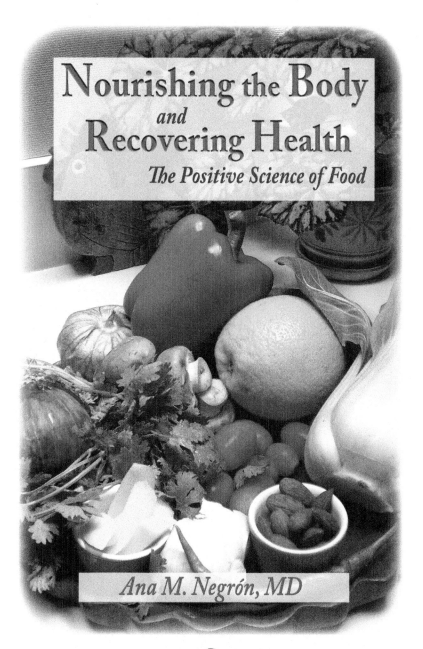

Nourishing the Body
and
Recovering Health
The Positive Science of Food

Ana M. Negrón, MD

Sunstone Press

SANTA FE

Sunstone books may be purchased for educational, business, or sales promotional use.
For information please write: Special Markets Department, Sunstone Press,
P.O. Box 2321, Santa Fe, New Mexico 87504-2321.

All photographs by Ana M. Negrón
Book and cover design › Vicki Ahl
Body typeface › Adobe Caslon Pro
Printed on acid-free paper
∞
eBook 978-1-61139-380-4

───

Library of Congress Cataloging-in-Publication Data

Negrón, Ana M., 1947-
Nourishing the body and recovering health : the positive science of food / by
Ana M. Negrón, MD.
    pages cm
Includes index.
    ISBN 978-1-63293-064-4 (softcover : alk. paper) -- ISBN 978-1-63293-065-1
(hardcover : alk. paper)
1. Nutrition. 2. Health. 3. Diet therapy. I. Title.
RA784.N44 2015
613.2--dc23
                                    2015010866

───

WWW.SUNSTONEPRESS.COM
SUNSTONE PRESS / POST OFFICE BOX 2321 / SANTA FE, NM 87504-2321 /USA
(505) 988-4418 / ORDERS ONLY (800) 243-5644 / FAX (505) 988-1025

Dedication

To my son, Jason Binnick, who believed I could write this book. To Trina Gelabert, my mom, who embodied it. To all of you who inspire me.

Contents

Foreword

*T*his book is your key to a healthier life. Its author, Ana M. Negrón, MD, is an exceptional physician. Not only is she thoroughly trained in state-of-the-art medical care; her knowledge and skills go several steps further, allowing her to show you how to maximize your health and tackle the fundamental causes of health problems that might be bothering you. If high blood pressure, diabetes, excess weight, or a high cholesterol level has its roots in eating habits that need an overhaul, Dr. Negrón will guide you to fixing the problem. Over the short run, that means feeling dramatically better. Over the long run, it means a revolution in your health, protecting you and your family against many problems down the road.

When I was in medical school, I was not prepared for the power that nutrition can have. In dealing with common health issues, we focused on medications, and we knew little about the healing power of foods. However, in recent years, a number of researchers have developed very powerful nutritional interventions, and the results are spectacular.

If you thought nutrition might do nothing more than helping you trim away a pound or two, or bringing cholesterol down a notch, you should know that nutrition's power goes well beyond that. Research studies by our team and others have shown that, with the power of good nutrition, you can reverse heart disease and diabetes, make weight problems improve dramatically, change how you look and feel, and even save your life.

This book puts that power to work. It will help you evaluate your kitchen with a virtual tour exercise, show you how to select the right foods, how to prepare them, and which foods you're better off without. It will even give you your own personal three-month guide to wellness through plant based nutrition. Dr. Negrón regularly cooks with her patients, so in the process, it will also show you how to save time and money. This book tackles the mental game, too—helping you deal with cravings, food addictions, and those little rationalizations that get in the way as we try to improve our health. As a bonus, you will find a section on common health conditions and the role that nutrition plays in causing them—and in curing them.

Board-certified in Family Medicine and equally expert in the science of nutrition, Dr. Negrón has helped countless people reclaim their health. Now she will help you, too. Let me encourage you to read this book thoroughly, put its guidance to work, and share what you have learned with your family and friends. In the process, you will pass along knowledge that will save lives. The journey is engaging, empowering, and fun.

I wish you the very best of health.

—Neal D. Barnard, MD, Adjunct Associate Professor of Medicine
George Washington University School of Medicine
President, Physicians Committee for Responsible Medicine
Washington, DC

Preface

Spring of 2003. It was Monday afternoon. My last patient needed refills for a cholesterol drug, a blood pressure pill, and two diabetes medications. She was only forty-two and would likely be on them for the rest of her life. Today she also wanted relief from acid reflux.

As I made my way back to the exam room with a new prescription pad (compliments of a pharmaceutical company), I began tearing out an ad every sixth page, for medications that promised to address each of my patient's conditions. I walked past the clinic pharmacy—always lit up like a supermarket.

For the first time in thirty years I had a visceral reaction as I put pen to the paper. I was the pathetic slave of a profit driven industry far from the medicine of my dreams watching the health and wellness of my patients slip away. Coming out of my trance I delivered her prescriptions and curiously felt my body relax.

Next Monday together with my stethoscope I brought a cooked sample of steel cut oats and quinoa mixed with plump blueberries. Colleagues were intrigued but didn't know what they tasted. The following week I brought a kale stir fry seasoned with garlic and lemon. Again: "This is delicious. What is it?"

I have my roots in *Diet For A New America* by John Robbins which opened my heart, but to my patients this nourishing plant food upon which I personally relied was life-giving non-prescription medicine. I recognized that without food literacy the admonition to *eat more vegetables* would remain merely a slogan. Then again, I was not a cook I am a physician. In spite of all this back and forth the genie would not go back in the bottle. What now?

That afternoon I found a brochure from the USDA's 5-A-Day program and Produce for Better Health Foundation in my mail box. Among advertisements for coloring books, plastic bananas, and toy shopping carts, it offered large 2 x 4 feet posters crammed with small colorful photographs of real fruits and vegetables. I ordered four and mounted them on foam board then hung one in each exam room. Patients stood inches from the wall studying the grid. Sometimes I felt I was interrupting deeply personal moments, that they were looking for an old friend in the crowd, or connecting to their ancestors.

My next step was inevitable. Armed with a dozen large cutting boards, a dozen sharp knives, a hot plate, and two gigantic stainless steel bowls, I scheduled cooking workshops. We alternated Spanish and English, expanded food literacy, added different fruits to our oats and an endless variety of ingredients to a savory rainbow salad. The cinnamon and cilantro aromas wafting into the hallways brought in many curious visitors. For two years and thanks to a generous couple I had the gift of a helper who came every month. The goal of the cooking sessions was and is to introduce tasty and nourishing food alternatives that would crowd out culprit items and help people recover from disease.

I noticed that few people regardless of the level of education knew leafy greens other than lettuce or spinach and scarcely any could name a whole grain other than rice. Folks would proudly repeat nutritional sound bites but couldn't defend them. It was then that I decided that no matter the type of audience, my lectures would always include sample foods. Excited to see patients reduce dependence on medications I was learning that this was scientifically expected, but few of my colleagues showed interest. This stung, yet came as no surprise. From my own experience I knew that studying this new way was an energy consuming challenge and that a change of attitude would take time.

In the early nineties I was lucky to find Physicians Committee for Responsible Medicine. Founded in 1985, PCRM promotes preventive medicine through nutrition, encourages higher standards in medical school education, and is shaping a new model of clinical research. I finally recognized them as my tribe and got ready to walk with them.

As I sought out independent studies with no ties to food or pharmaceutical industries, I kept finding mountains of evidence for the arrest and reversal not just for heart disease but for most chronic illnesses that plague western countries. So began the most laborious and satisfying phase of my medical career and I was not alone. I restudied biochemistry and physiology, formally learned the role of food in medicine, sought mentoring, pored over clinical research, collated tables and references, created recipes, wrote essays, compiled healthy suggestions, and in 2008 with the help of my son, Jason Binnick, we designed www.greensonabudget.org which still houses my work in progress.

When in the past people prompted me to write a book my response was always that I was living it. My thanks to all of you who watered this seed. Today I want to share its fruit with you.

Introduction

$\mathcal{T}$his book is an antidote to our chronic reliance on pharmaceuticals. It presents basic nutrition information expanding it with more sophisticated medical discussions, so whether you are beginning to explore plant foods or an experienced student of food in medicine, it was written for you.

This book is a guide to better health and wellness through excellent nourishment. It recommends foods with an all around excellent nutritional profile and does not chase after single ingredients, thereby helping you avoid marketing traps. Some might reproach not finding hot topics like genetically modified crops (GMOs), organic meats, or honey from wild bees; I urge you to make personal informed decisions. If you are curious why this book does not endorse detoxification programs and other gimmicks or if you look in vain for comments on current fads, keep these general principles in mind: Plant foods are good-for-you and processed and animal foods are not-so-good for you. The only supplement we should all be taking is Vitamin B_{12}.

This book strives to make health care a simple and affordable personal responsibility. As a result we will need less sick care. It presents complicated topics in simple terms and celebrates the stories of real people. It covers basic nutrition, body literacy, and more than twenty medical conditions. Although I have been told that the average person does not care about references, I hope they are wrong. By referring to actual research questions and the current body of scientific evidence, we will not drift at the mercy of opinions or those who promulgate them. I encourage you to visit credible sources and shape your own.

My mission is to show some of the body's inner workings and reveal the intimate relationship we have with food, our only source of nourishment. I try to remove obstacles, such as perhaps a lack of familiarity with foods or a cluttered kitchen environment. I do away with harmful nutrition myths and clear misunderstandings regarding the cost, time, and effort needed to nourish oneself well. My hope is to remind us that these amazing bodies we inhabit are willing to go the distance.

We pay dearly for favoring a pill over prevention. It is astonishing the number of people who suffer from a poor diet and excess weight. In the U.S. as of 2014 around 25 million people have diabetes; 26 million suffer from asthma; 40 million have painful arthritis; 60 million have irritable bowel; more than 60 million suffer from acid reflux; 65 million have high blood pressure; 78 million adults and almost 13 million young are obese; and 90 million live constipated.

Hooked on big pharma, each year Americans spend over 200 billion dollars on prescription medications (up from the equivalent of 22 billion in 1960) and an additional 25 to 30 billion in supplements and other over the counter drugs. For example, Viagra a blockbuster drug for Pfizer and marketed for erectile dysfunction has annual U.S. sales of $1.2 billion.

Every year since 1985 when direct pharmaceutical advertising to consumers became legal in the United States billions of dollars poured into this form of marketing. At the end of their patent, many prescription drugs find their way into the booming world of over the counter medications.

Adding more drugs to diabetes has not stopped the disease. Despite ten classes of blood pressure medications, heart attacks remain the number one killer. The U.S. and Northern Europe (where there is ample access to bone building drugs) have the highest hip fracture rates compared to the lowest rates in Latin America and Africa. Although the U.S. spends more on health care than any of the other top seven industrialized countries in the world, it ranks last on gross national health. We focus on combatting our burgeoning diseases while we ignore prevention.

Consider these contradictions. We need around 2000 calories a day, yet the United States produces around 3900 calories per person per day (mostly from animal and factory foods). These excess 1900 calories are linked to obesity, high lipids, high sugars, high blood pressure, heart disease, and cancers, whereas a shift to eating less and mostly plant foods would help us need less sick care. It is ironic that in this land of plenty the United States Department of Agriculture (USDA) reports that Americans eat less than the recommended amount of fruits and vegetables—highly nutritious foods naturally low in calories, which could satisfy all our requirements.

Here is another dissonant note. The poor in the U.S. (and in other developed countries) are disproportionately affected by obesity and chronic illness. Whole plant foods represent non prescription medicine that can help us reclaim health, so why do we funnel unsold baked goods to local needy organizations for the poor? As an example, in 2010 a bakery-cafe with 1700 locations throughout the country reportedly donated a retail value worth about $100 million of their products made from flour, sugar, oil, and salt, contributing thousands of hardly nutritious extra calories to vulnerable populations. I watch donor trucks unload breads, huge bagels, pizzas, cakes, and pies, at senior centers as patrons wobble to pick up their share.

As we continue to speculate on how we got here, we sink deeper into obesity and its consequences. Our landscape is dotted with countless outlets for fast food: MacDonald's 14,000; Subway 24,000; Pizza Hut 6,000; Burger King 7,500; Taco Bell 5,000, Wendy's 5,000. Their edibles—made in large factories using electricity, running water, specialized machinery, and skilled operators—sell cheaper than fresh produce.

Television dedicates two network channels (Food Network and Cooking Channel) solely to cooking. In 2014 they announced adding 35 more cooking shows. If while surfing the channels you land on one of these 200+ shows you will be treated to the oohs and aahs of fat and sugar. Scheduled programing confirms a total disregard for health and nutrition. Popular reality television shows follow people struggling with pounds. Tabloids portray stars in endless weight cycles. A famous TV chef (her weakness is sugar and fat) announces she has diabetes. A beloved actor dies of a heart attack at fifty-one.

Athletes sing the praises of arthritis medicines; politicians normalize the use of pills for sexual function; we sign on to a milk mustache for strong bones; a purple pill for relief for heartburn, and daily yogurt for irritable bowel. We forget that these ads represent the interests of for profit industry playing us like puppets. We are again won over by a figment magic bullet that we hope could solve our problems.

Knowledge is power. However, we will use it when we are ready. At eighty-six my mom finally traded the bland colors of chicken, bread, crackers, cheese, and mayonnaise for the rainbow colors of strawberries, grapefruit, melon, broccoli, pumpkin, sprouts, lentils, and sweet potato. She was surprised that within a month her body responded with more elasticity, less pain, more energy, and a sharper mind. Her only regret was not starting sooner. Be assured that any time is soon enough.

Herein lies perhaps the biggest obstacle to the simple practice of health care: although we are suffering diseases of excess and not of deprivation, we are conditioned to see ourselves as lacking. Think of the ads that permeate our environment reminding us how we lack beauty, youth, hair, money, or sex appeal. The general perception is that we also lack vitamins, calcium, good fats, and protein, so we can't imagine how using less of anything could be good for us. The simple elimination of animal and factory foods to regain health seems unsophisticated, yet regarding diseases of excess it is just the thing to do. Removing these obstacles gets us closer to wellness.

Adults, not children, hold the purse. We cannot act surprised that we have spread the obesity epidemic to our young. If they are overfed and malnourished, the burden is on us. This problem needs more than a signed piece of legislation. Around 2003, an Arkansas governor lost more than one hundred pounds for health reasons. As a result of his personal experience he discovered that the obesity epidemic was also affecting children, so he decided to raise awareness of the situation and decreed that schools send home the child's body mass index—BMI tracks height and weight adjusted for age and sex. Unfortunately his measure (which became law in Arkansas and was adopted in twenty other states), lacked substantial initiatives that could reverse the obesity trend. The school cafeterias still serve high fat and sugar foods, children have shrinking gym and recess time, and the staff walks the halls as overweight as the student body, which points to a systemic problem. (Incidentally the governor regained his weight.)

Even under the most recent Childhood Nutrition Act, schools continue to serve fast food, such as pizza, burgers, nuggets, cheese sticks with ketchup plus sweet flavored milk. Tasteless "fresh" fruit and baby carrots come out of bags in the refrigerator. No school should receive kudos because burgers are now served on whole wheat buns or because nuggets are baked instead of fried. Such meager cosmetic changes numb our resolve to do better.

This book aims to inspire the use of delicious plant food for sustenance, disease prevention, and often cure. Simple recipes and photos prompt you to make durable changes in your nutrition. Those interested in science will find sections which stimulate a more in depth reading on biochemistry and physiology. Parents will learn how to involve the family with effective, evidence based practical suggestions. You will read about people in progress and not just success stories.

Our current generation of teens and preteens is using over the counter drugs for the relief of headaches, acid stomachs, general malaise, and aches. They use energy drinks to combat fatigue, lack of focus, and depression. These patterns are getting established early and will be hard to change. Schools are where children spend much of their time and are in the position to implement a sensory based comprehensive nutrition education as the rule rather than the exception.

At the other end of the age spectrum, seniors are considered set in their ways no longer able to benefit from a healthier diet. We have accepted deterioration and disease as part of growing old, yet nothing could be further from the truth. With nourishing food the body will quickly recover to the extent possible. At any age we can retrain our taste buds. If a medication altered the savoring ability and hurting or missing teeth impaired chewing, these should be addressed rather than endured. While people are entitled to chose what they want to eat, elder havens should not serve comfort food regardless of nutritional value. Serving ham and buttered mashed potatoes, pasta with meatballs, pork loin, cheese macaroni, marshmallow sweet potatoes, fried chicken, bread, juice, brownies, cake, and ice cream, to people with diabetes, hypertension, heart disease, arthritis, and Alzheimer's is indefensible. Low cost meals can and should be nourishing.

The western model of medicine is without par when dealing with infections, broken bones, and surgical emergencies, but it is woefully inadequate when applied to chronic diseases like diabetes and heart disease. Rare conditions such as hemophilia, Huntington's chorea, or Tay Sachs are truly determined by inheritance, but for most diseases our genes function like blueprints. We don't need to develop a disease just because we have the manual. People from countries where obesity, diabetes, and heart disease are rare, develop them within a few years of adopting the typical American diet, that is the bad news. The good news is that science bursts at the seams with evidence that this process is reversible. Although diseases are observed to run in families, the switch that turns many disease genes on and off can be kept idle by eating mostly nourishing foods and no more than necessary. Developments in the field of epigenetics support the notion that we can protect ourselves from arthritis, hypertension, diabetes, heart disease, sexual dysfunction, and many cancers, on excellent nutrition and a healthy lifestyle.

In the 1990s Dean Ornish demonstrated that heart disease can be arrested and even reversed with a program consisting of low fat plant based foods, exercise, and meditation. His discovery is now accepted by mainstream medicine and is growing in breadth and depth. Eminent scientists and progressive clinicians like Caldwell Esselstyn, John McDougall, Neal Barnard, Joel Fuhrman, and many others continue to advance the role of plant food for our protection and in the treatment of disease. T. Colin Campbell's *The China Study* published in 2004, gives ample evidence that chronic disease correlates with the consumption of animal products.

People who live hectic lives often don't want to cook. Deciding what's for dinner at the last minute restricts one to microwave and take out, where healthful choices are few and boring. This also means that the average American kitchen is not stocked to meet the family's nutritional needs. Not cooking creates a huge problem. The main goal of having recipes in this book is to bring you willingly into the kitchen to show that time, energy, and money are not obstacles. People who feel alone and unsupported could invite others to cook with them and build up each others' food bank. To those who are parents, I remind you that children who are introduced the kitchen early and in a friendly manner grow to be food literate adults with life saving cooking skills. This is a priceless legacy.

Even with the Affordable Care Act (Obamacare) fifty million Americans are still without health insurance and many more are without a drug plan, yet no one needs insurance to adopt a more healing lifestyle. This book encourages you to seek out help from physicians, nurse practitioners, dietitians, food literate friends, mentors who can guide you. Find inspiration in this author's ongoing program cooking with patients and their families. (See Greens on a Budget, and Recipes.)

Advertisements often focus on a product's one redeeming quality, yet we should choose foods with an all around excellent profile. This way collard greens win over milk because they have large amount of usable calcium, protect us with carotenes, sulforaphanes, fiber, and vitamin C, plus have none of the risks associated with dairy (such as cancers, osteoporosis, and acne).

Our diet is linked to the highest cost of health care in the world. You may feel frustrated that administrators and politicians drag their feet or demand always more research before changing bad policies; remember that they are influenced by special interests. This country pays a high ethical price slaughtering ten billion animals for food every year; no one needs permission to eat less animals and more plants. Be part of the change you want. Practice wellness where you are. Cook, walk, cycle, dance. If you are a smoker quit. We may not be able to avoid an accident, leave a stressful job, change our economic status, abandon where we live, or change the air we breathe, but through excellent nutrition we can live healthier lives with less drugs or their side effects.

"I can explain it to you, but I cannot comprehend it for you."
—Ed Koch, Mayor of New York

Part I

Personal Guide to Health

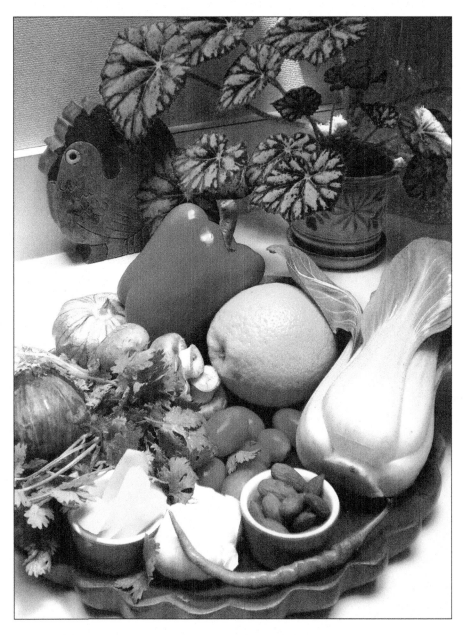

On the day you are cooking, group the ingredients for each recipe. Viewed in context, their array of colors, textures, aromas, and evoked flavors will inspire you to experiment with other vegetables and different combinations.

1

Experience the Positive Science of Food

For a growing number of you this is a refresher course affirming the wellness practices of good nourishment, exercise, meditation, and self expression. For others the weeks ahead could chart the new direction you were longing for, the new path you are ready to take. Perhaps this time the challenge is to stay on your wellness practice for longer than ever before. Even for life.

The vast majority of chronic diseases which plague our developed world are not external attacks, but the result of not regularly tending to our health and wellbeing. We have exposed the body to an excess of processed and animal foods and not enough to whole foods for the body to thrive. We can take this back.

If you have been on a frequent dose of chicken, bread, cheese, fish, juice, boxed cereals, pizza, fritters, sweets, and take out, it is likely that you are also on medicines for conditions such as arthritis, pain, high cholesterol, high blood pressure, diabetes, heart disease, sexual dysfunction, acid reflux, allergies, asthma, depression, irritable bowel, and constipation.

The above foods produce inflammation, make our blood viscous, raise blood pressure, and elevate blood lipids. The body suffers with increased fat stores, insulin resistance, and foods that stimulate uncontrolled cell division. Deep inside we already know this.

If you could, be still for a couple of minutes and tune in to your body. Hear its constant hum: heart pumping, hair growing, gastric juices pouring into the stomach, cuts and bruises healing, nourishment from the latest meal being absorbed into the bloodstream, insulin carrying sugar into muscles and brain, excess fat being removed from inside arteries, liver, and underneath your skin, inflammation turning on and off appropriately, dying red blood cells replaced by new ones, bacteria being zapped, rogue cancer cells biting the dust. Feel intestines pushing their load, oxygenation and pH carefully monitored. You sense not just the temperature but also the atmosphere and mood in the room. Marvel that you are, you've come this far; relax, let go of stress, and stay alert.

Trust that food is positive medicine: As you switch to a daily dose of kale, collards, squash, potato, oats, quinoa, beans, rice, berries, mango, broccoli, cauliflower, daikon, and Swiss chard, you begin to lose many symptoms and your need for medications. Sustain life functions by eating an abundance of whole plant foods loaded with vitamins, phytochemicals, antioxidants, cancer protection, fiber, and anti-inflammatory chemicals—top-of-the-line raw materials for the body to carry out its magic.

Invest in yourself. Imagine trading some old habits for new ones. Set a plan in motion. Use the next few weeks to develop a new attitude toward your well being. Acknowledge that the greatest challenge is to sustain a wellness practice. Plan for success.

As better foods replace the more standard diet, your body begins to flush out toxins and you will feel out of sorts for two or three days—more sleepy, perhaps get a headache, or grumbling in the stomach. Take notice, but don't panic. As you transition, your intestines will be the first to wake up.

Depending on your cravings you will have withdrawals. Accept it, do not get your fix of cheese, or meat, or sugar. Record changes in your mood, in your body, in your energy, in your appreciation for all life. This is your experience.

Surrender to the process. By the end of the first week you lose a few pounds of water, which were held by inflammation and your skin feels more alive. Aches start to dissipate, you are more agile, your step has a bounce, you no longer have acid reflux, your blood pressure is dropping, your sugars are normalizing, your triglycerides are going down. The impact of your new lifestyle will take many forms and will continue to be felt in the months and years to come as your experience unfolds.

Remember that no matter our age, no matter our condition, we wake up newer every day. Tonight, simply rest well.

2

Start With Six Weeks

*A*lthough this chapter makes the case for transitioning to a healthier lifestyle, it introduces it as a plan to be tried for six weeks with the option of extending it to three months, six months, a year, and beyond. Americans waste billions of dollars a year on diets. I say waste, because most people do not keep the weight off after the diet, so they may repeat the same one again or try a new one. On the other hand, people who transition to a healthier lifestyle waste less money and often manage to stick with it.

Eating nourishing plant foods will help you lose excess weight and restores health to its fullest potential. However, your new habits must stand in stark contrast with your old ones. Wimpy efforts don't pay off and will leave you disappointed. The changes here suggested are profound.

Test this lifestyle for a minimum of six weeks: Plan to eliminate culprit foods. Do not play mind games by reducing them. Even if you don't plan to keep going beyond six weeks, give this experiment your all. Be living proof that when you treat your body well, it will go the distance. After six weeks you could choose either to live a healthier life or go back, but your choice will be based on true personal experience.

Many symptoms such as acid reflux, joint aches, bloating, and trouble sleeping, will go away early on, but in six weeks you will significantly improve health parameters such as blood pressure, blood sugar, and lipids.

Prepare for change, this is not a diet. This is the way to reclaim as much lost health as you possibly can. Read on, imagine how you can positively make it work.

TIMETABLE

The plan begins with a ten day pilot which extends
to a minimum of six weeks:

Pilot: three days plus seven for a total of ten days.

After the pilot:
Day one
Week one
Six weeks
Three months
Six months
One year
Beyond

GETTING READY TO START

Pick a suitable day within a month and mark it on your calendar. On such day you will start eliminating some foods replacing them with more nourishing ones. In essence you will be breaking long established food habits. This will demand your full attention, so be sure you can rest, perhaps take a few days off, get a sitter if you need one, cancel meetings.

Gather your kitchen tools, enlist any help you might require, be disciplined, plan to work hard and not give up for at least six weeks. If you hire a chef or buy prepared food, you will miss an integral part of this plan. The act of preparing a meal is in itself transforming.

Don't juggle all at once. Pace yourself, select a few simple recipes (you can choose some from this book) and cook them in advance. For example: a pot of oats and quinoa; a pot of rice; a pot of beans; a fruit salad; a leafy rainbow salad.

If you are just getting to know whole plants or feel shy about using new ingredients you may want to consult with a professional. Work with someone who uses whole plants for nourishment and ideally also applies this to his or her life. Depending on your expertise in the kitchen and your food literacy, one or two consulting sessions at the beginning might prove enough. Schedule a refresher within a reasonable agreed time to keep growing.

PILOT

Begin with a short trial of three days during which you will check if your projections regarding time to shop, prep, and cook are reasonable. Then give yourself seven more days to fix obvious glitches. Record new or surprising experiences.

THE VIRTUAL KITCHEN TOUR EXERCISE

I find that food diaries render incomplete stories of the way we eat, in part because memory of past events tends to be selective. I have also found that diet histories can be fudged. For example, we might unconsciously forget foods about which we feel guilty or perhaps include healthier foods we plan to eat, but haven't yet. In contrast, during a virtual kitchen tour the person tries to visualize the food that is in the house at the moment—I call this our food bank. Even if most meals are not consumed at home the Virtual Kitchen Tour could give us a head start on improving our nutrition balance.

This exercise is best done in pairs between family members or friends: one person recalls and one takes notes then they switch roles. A sheet of stickers will come in handy for the second half of the exercise when you will tag some foods before deciding what to do with them.

RULES

1. Whether you recently went shopping or plan to go in the next couple of days, just get on with it.
2. Avoid any comments, judgements, or explanations during the exercise. Stay focused on the task.
3. Be quick and objective as you gather the details. Ten minutes is usually enough time.

FIRST PART

Procedure:

1. Systematically recall all food and drink within the house today, while your exercise partner jots it down.
2. Begin with kitchen counters then refrigerator, freezer, pantry, cupboards, and any other place where food is stashed, such as special cabinets, basement freezer, or overflow storage.
3. Include soda, juice, energy drinks, and alcohol. Include oils, flours, sugars; note the size of the containers and how often they are

replenished. (Condiments will be discussed in Chapter 14, "A Well Stocked Kitchen.") Be sure to ask about bread, boxed cereal, and snack items, such as granola, candy, chocolate, pretzels, chips, and so called energy bars. Don't forget deli meats, cheese, left overs, and ice cream. Ask about bottled water, money misspent on this commodity is often taken away from the food budget.

Now switch positions with your partner and complete the exercise before reading on.

Note foods you mentioned first and note foods that you omitted. This could mean that you have assigned them either special positive or negative value.

Later you can refer to chapter 14, A Well Stocked Kitched, and do just that. Continue making adjustments. Clearly state your goals: to be better nourished, to lose weight, to stop a disease, to depend less on medications, and so on. Then refine them: to delight in caring for my body, to love the way I eat; to make this my lifestyle; and so on. Every now and then take a fresh look at your kitchen and redress noted imbalances.

SECOND PART

This part of the exercise asks you to identify non plant foods in your kitchen. Affix a red sticker to every processed food on your list (concentrate on packages with more than one ingredient). You will find this visual image helpful as you later begin to correct imbalances. If processed boxed and canned goods dominate your kitchen, you are not alone.

I suggest you examine the red sticker items in your kitchen. Start by eliminating anything that you need to ration, lock up, or hide. This is especially important for children, but also helps adults. Discover how to satisfy hunger with healthy food and model it for the young ones.

After going on hundreds of virtual kitchen tours I find a dearth of plant foods. About seventy-five percent of kitchens I visit have no leafy greens other than lettuce, spinach, or a bag of spring mix. Most sport the same few specimens of plants: carrots, celery, cucumbers, bananas, apples, grapes, and oranges. If any grains, it is mostly rice, microwave popcorn, and instant oats. The most common legume is peanut, usually as peanut butter. Beets, sweet potatoes, and other roots are usually absent. Pumpkins decorate the stoop on Halloween.

We all shop based on habit and taste preferences, so there are no set answers, merely starting points that invite learning. The kitchen mirrors our nutrition even if we don't always eat in. As you do this exercise the task of balancing your nutrition becomes clearer.

Ask yourself these questions and gain even more insight:

1. How often do you cook? Do others in the home also cook?
2. How comfortable, well lit, and uncluttered is your kitchen?
3. How would you describe your cooking space and counter tops?
4. How large is your chopping board? Does it need maintenance such as oiling?
5. What size is your vegetable knife and how do you sharpen it?
6. What vegetables and leafy greens are in your refrigerator today?
7. How many home cooked meals are in the freezer right now?
8. What do you offer your guests to eat? To drink?
9. Where and how often do you buy fresh produce? How far is it from your home or office?
10. What can you say about organic foods?
11. How much do you pay for a pound of rice? oats? beans?
12. What do you buy in cans?
13. What condiments do you use?
14. Name your breads: bagel, tortilla, pizza, muffin, pretzel, cookies, crackers.
15. What size container of oil do you buy? How often do you replenish it?
16. Where do you sit down to eat your meals?
17. What will you have for dinner tonight?
18. Name places where you go out to eat. What are your favorite items on the menu? Where do you go for take out?

PREPARING FOR DAY ONE

Complete the above VIRTUAL KITCHEN TOUR and deal with some of the sticker items. Get ready to replace meat, cheese, oil, sweets, and baked goods with a nourishing menu like the one below. Cook in advance: a pot of rice, a pot of beans, bake some vegetables, and make a soup. Take photos of your face and hands. You will be comparing them in three weeks.

Think before shopping for too many ingredients, this is usually wasteful. You will clutter the kitchen and much of it will spoil since you won't be able to use it all. Don't shop hungry or without a list. Use a couple of recipes as guide and buy only what you need.

Be aware that as you replace meat, cheese, and processed items with whole plant foods you are in a dynamic transformation, so you might get a headache, come down with a cold, experience loose stools, or feel really tired. Remain active, but get enough rest. Drink plenty of water. Eat your nourishing meals. Stay alert. Study your hunger. Above all do not misinterpret these symptoms as needing the foods you left behind.

DAY ONE

You have been preparing for this adventure. This is your first day. Whatever brought you here must be worth going through with it. Give it your all. The goal of these six weeks is to develop a new habit in service of your health, not to be amused with a different recipe every day, so stick to the basic menu. Enjoy variety by using different fruits in your oats or different leafy greens for your stir fry. Consult the recipes and photos in this book.

A SAMPLE DAY

Breakfast: Cook oats and quinoa in cinnamon and water. Add fruit when done then sprinkle with ground flax seed. It will sustain you all morning.

Snack: A medley of diced fresh fruit.

Lunch: Stir fry garlic and onion with a teaspoon of oil in the skillet, add a cup each of diced (half inch cubes) squash and tomatoes, slice another cup of mushrooms and radishes, add a few tablespoons of cooked brown rice and a few tablespoons of cooked beans (or several slices of tofu or tempeh). In 10 minutes the vegetables will be tender soft. Add four cups of chopped leafy greens and season with your choice of spices, salt and pepper, and cover for 5 more minutes. You will have enough for a few servings without worrying about the calories.

Snack: Mix shredded carrots into humus and scoop with slices of kohlrabi; or perhaps wrap a lemon drizzled wedge of avocado in a Napa cabbage leaf.

Dinner: Enjoy a slice of whole grain bread with a cup of vegetable soup (onion, garlic, diced sweet potato, broccoli, carrot, corn, mushrooms, plus four cups of chopped leafy greens like collards, bok choy, or Asian mustard greens).

Evening Snack: Finish the day with any bit of your day's left overs or a fruit medley topped with a couple of nuts.

Drink enough water. If you drink stimulants like coffee or tea, limit them to a cup a day; if you drink alcohol, limit it to a glass of wine a day. More could upset the new balance of your gastrointestinal system.

THE FIRST WEEK AND BEYOND

If you are working with a consultant, after a weekend and five weekdays would be a good time to check in and bring up any questions. If you are otherwise comfortable, repeat the same menu for a few more weeks. Tweak your new recipes, but keep them simple. You are using foods and techniques that might be new to you, so focus on establishing a new habit. Variety will come later. Stay grounded.

Again take photos of your hands and face. How do they compare with the ones you took three weeks earlier? You may notice that much of the puffiness is gone.

The contrast between old and new habits must be clear, this cannot be stressed enough. Make profound changes and stick to them. If you insist on just reducing some foods or eating them less often, you have done that exact thing before and the results were disappointing.

Within the first month of eliminating culprit foods, joint aches, acid reflux, constipation, and bloating will melt away. Enjoy the glow on your face. You will have more energy and will be less dependent on prescription drugs. Exercise. It will feel good to dance, walk, or swim, just move.

Soon you are into week six and feeling more comfortable planning and shopping. Cooking begins to find a rhythm. A stash of home cooked meals is growing in the freezer. You are savoring new foods. You feel lighter and more confident, more at home in your body. A world of plant foods is opening up and you are better nourished.

Since benefits accrue over time, you may decide to go on for another six weeks, which brings you to three months.

THE FIRST THREE MONTHS

You have less inflammation as whole plant foods help mop up and eliminate toxins. Avoid discomfort from sudden increases in fiber by eating small portions of new plant foods. Occasionally you may be tired, feel a grumbling in the stomach, or get a headache. Slow down or rest, but don't go back.

You have lost weight if that was one of your goals plus blood lipids, blood sugar, and blood pressure may all be normal. If you have been consistent in recording your experiences, revisit them now after three months. Any surprises?

ANOTHER THREE MONTHS

You may decide to give yourself three more months and then another three. Experience the subtle ripples of wellness and health. Although some benefits will be palpable in the short run, they will continue to unfold over a lifetime.

THE FIRST YEAR

Before you know it, you have lived a year in more health and wellness. Some people continue to make journal entries or take photos of their bodies. Remember the symptoms which first brought you to make changes, keep the commitment alive.

Care for your body. Listen to it through every year cycle. Occasionally you may need to restart, but never abandon the work.

FAD DIETS

We humans live in perennial tension between total freedom and self control. We are not great at negotiating this balance, that is why we create laws, but with practice we are meant to use our own set of internal checks and balances. That is how we exercise free will responsibly.

Fad diets promise weight loss with ready made rules and prohibitions, but they don't educate about food or about the body's nourishment needs. This is how millions get lost in the up and down of pounds lost and regained. Weight swings of twenty pounds or more increase the risk of gall stone formation—a fact which stresses the web of interconnections within the body. Diets are some of the longest short cuts in the world.

HELPFUL HINTS

Once you understand your body's metabolic rhythm you won't have to be forever watching your weight. Begin by getting on the scale every day for two weeks then once a week for two months. Write the weights down, don't skip this step. Notice small variations up and down; spot trends. Do not obsess, but use this exercise to understand how your body handles what you eat. Correct small deviations with portions or type of foods. Soon you will be able to tell your weight by how you feel, by the reflection in a mirror, or by the fit of your clothes. Be mindful of the calorie spread in your diet: aim for 70% carbohydrates, 10% protein, and no more than 20% fat. A diet composed of a variety of whole plant foods will have a balanced distribution of these nutrients. We will talk about this later. When you feel ready, give up the scale and check your weight just every now and then. Enjoy eating healthfully.

3

Make New Habits

LET GO OLD HABITS: If you are already on medications, they are suppressing symptoms but not restoring your health. If your nutritional imbalance has been chipping away at your wellbeing, it is time to make a change. Think of replacing foods such as meat, cheese, baked goods, sweets, and oils, with abundant nutritious whole plant foods. Simply cutting back or adding a few plants is not enough, especially if you are already sick. Once you recover you are in better position to decide how or whether to reintroduce any culprit foods into your diet.

Besides lacking wholeness and many nutrients, factory foods (processed and packaged items usually made with sugars, flours, and/or oils), promote inflammation by generating disproportionate amounts of free radicals. Among young people, the enormous amount of refined ingredients embedded in these foods have replaced nourishing whole foods. There are no new ingredients on the shelves, only new combinations.

The human body lives in a dynamic equilibrium—support it. Eliminate sweet drinks and drink only water. Record how soon your taste buds become sensitive to the natural sugars in plants. The time may be shorter than you expect. In a similar way, taste buds adjust to less fat and the same goes for salt. Put your senses to the test.

MAKE NEW HABITS: We know of people (perhaps even ourselves) who've made radical changes, abruptly and completely or as they say cold turkey. At the sight of his first born daughter my dad quit smoking. At eighty-six my mom went plant based and felt younger. Some people survive a heart attack or a bout of cancer and embark on surprising adventures, often in their own backyards. What might compel a couch potato to take out the old tennis racket and head for the court? What moves the lifetime homemaker to start a business? Why would the retired teacher take swimming lessons? What is it that clicks making us feel fully alive? At least ten times you have altered the course of your life. How did it happen? How did you do it?

According to the *New Oxford American Dictionary* a habit is: a settled or regular tendency or practice, especially one that is hard to give up. Habits are semiconscious acts. Some are innocent and inconsequential such as putting on pants right leg first, others like shopping for the same food items each week could be revised, but when we hang on to habits which are flat out harmful such as smoking, or which have outlived their usefulness like eating the greasy cafeteria food of when we were students, we stay in a dangerous rut. Replacing drugs with nourishing foods involves changing habits.

Thoughtful planning can make old habits easier to replace. Refrigerate several cooked dishes that can be mixed and matched with various greens throughout the week. This is not all you must do, but it is a healthy start.

Many delicious tasting foods await your acquaintance. (See Recipes.) Imagine yourself at work popping the lid to the aroma of a home cooked meal—not yet available at any snack bar or deli.

For example:

Collard greens with onion curry and a slice of corn bread; Brown rice with braised kale and beans in vegetable broth; Spicy arugula salad with pomegranate seeds.

Instead of yogurt, a cup of blueberries mixed with cooked quinoa and amaranth; slices of kohlrabi to scoop your guacamole; shredded carrot folded in humus with crunchy broccoli and cauliflower instead of chips; hot soup of pumpkin, sweet potato, and cashews.

Savory grains infused with lemon juice and cilantro. You've never had rice taste so good.

Seasoned baked beets or baked potato rounds or sweet potato sticks; refreshing cucumber or ginger water.

4

Relationships

*A*s you make necessary changes in your lifestyle and adapt your environment for a healthier body, you'll need to consider those around you. Here are some tips.

ADULTS

Most of us live with or around other people and our styles affect each other. Describe your plan in a sensitive manner, negotiate how to share the kitchen, and live in peace.

YOUNG CHILDREN

It is easy to engage children in a project. It is in their nature to be curious. Explain that the family will be learning about new foods, but keep it simple. When out food shopping, give them strips of colored cardboard and ask them to find produce of matching white, green, red, orange, and yellow. When you get home, draw and write the name of the fruit or vegetable on the card then read something about it.

Invite children into the kitchen. Their little fingers can rip up cabbage leaves, peel garlic and onion, pluck grapes from their stem, and push buttons on the blender. Combine food literacy and art. While you cook, let them glue pictures with different color dry grains and legumes. Sign their names with small seeds such as sesame, poppy, or chia. Find projects within their abilities: they can pit dates, stuff them with pomegranate seeds, or make a fruit tart of sliced fruit pressed on a raw pasty crust of nuts and dates. Teach them to rinse leafy greens in a bowl of cool water until they feel no more sand at the bottom. Exercise their imagination. Have them collect plant seeds from kitchen fruits and vegetables then plant them on the ground (label the spot) to see if they germinate. Before soaking beans, spread them on a towel and charge your child with picking out any tooth cracking pebbles. I keep a collection of them on a tiny shelf in the kitchen. Make sure your children grow up with rich whole food memories.

OLDER ADOLESCENTS

Teens are busy asserting their independence and forging alliances outside the home. However, as parents we must expose them among other things to nourishing food and it is our responsibility to teach them how to budget for the day they go live on their own. Show them these paragraphs.

Cash in on the relationship you have with your adolescent. As a member of the family he or she is already helping with some chores, add cooking to the list. Teach your teen to follow a written recipe all the way to serving the meal. Being able to cook is a skill that will serve him or her for a lifetime.

Accept suggestions. If you must show disapproval do it with respect never mockery. Let your child come up with a family meal and let him prepare it without supervision.

Your teen already knows how to call for pizza. Ask her to stop at the grocery store and pick up a few items that will expand her food literacy (such as butternut squash, collards, short brown rice, or capers). Challenge him to bring a bag of chips with less than 20% of the calories from fat or a bag of roasted chestnuts (the only nut low in fat) and read about them together.

Assign individuals to chop and dice the ingredients in advance (onions, garlic, red peppers, carrots, napa cabbage, and more) for the recipes of that week. As long as the task is finished the night before you plan to cook, let them do it on their own time. Leave the empty containers and written instructions on the counter. The day you cook fill up the same containers with individual portions for the freezer and the lunch box.

Remember, as adults we hold the purse. Don't let yourself be bullied into junk food.

FRIENDS AND WORKPLACE

Your changing lifestyle may not find unconditional support everywhere you go. Stay grounded. The office brings together people with diverse habits, values, and customs. Contribute to the healthy mix. Conserve your energies by not getting into pointless arguments. What you do will not suit everyone.

OPINIONS ARE NOT FACTS

Use the many references within this book to evaluate others' opinions as well as your own.

PREPARING FOOD WITH OTHERS

The kitchen is a focal point in a home. Share it beyond the usual tasks of setting the table or washing the dishes. Plan cooking time with family and friends. Teach children grown up tasks, like how to measure ingredients and how to follow a recipe. Teach them how to safely use a knife around other people.

Here's a fruit salad that is good for starters and everyone can participate.

INGREDIENTS: A couple of pineapples, ruby red grapefruits, apples, pears, grapes, and any other fruit in season like pomegranate, persimmons, plums, mangos, or melons.

MATERIALS: Have chopping boards and knives for each adult and older child; bowls for the young ones (they can fill them with plucked grapes or collect chopped fruit from around the table). Each task is important.

METHOD: Cube the fruit in uniform pieces about the size of grapes. Mix all the fruit using a generous size bowl at least 15 inches across. Refrigerate in small containers for packed lunches.

VARIATIONS: Add a personal touch to each serving: ground flax seeds, lemon juice, crushed nuts, a dollop of soy yogurt, or thinly sliced dates.

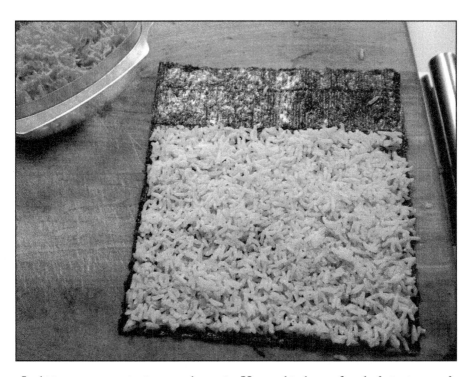

Sushi in progress—rice is a popular grain. Here a thin layer of cooked rice is spread on a nori seaweed sheet awaiting colorful matchsticks of vegetables such as carrots, red peppers, and thin wedges of avocado, before it is rolled into a log and sliced to one and a half inch rounds.

5

Food Savvy Children

*A*dults are in charge and must take full responsibility for the child's nutrition. A five year old who wants fast food is too young to know that her taste buds have been highjacked. Keep healthful delicious finger foods in the house (such as cherry tomatoes, dates, grapes, and radishes); avoid snacks that must be rationed (like soda, ice cream, candy, cookies, and chips), they will be coveted more; present nutritious foods with confidence and not as a tentative experiment that you believe might fail. Try new recipes with the family. Don't preach. Teach by example. Solicit comments, but don't give in or give up.

Today the Internet offers an encyclopedia at our fingertips enabling us to learn about different ingredients whenever we wish. Consult books such as *Plant Powered Diet, The Life Long Lasting Plan For Achieving Optimal Health Beginning Today* by Sharon Palmer, RD, 2012, The Experiment.

Discuss how food habits affect the economy of the family. Add up how much you spend on fast food and take out. Add up how much money goes to buy party food (such as sodas, bottled drinks, chips, and candy bars). Compare this with what you spend on more nutritious food. Are you wasting money on bottled water?

Explore the connection between common symptoms (like constipation, stomach pains, acid reflux, headaches, fatigue) and a poor diet. Your adolescent may be interested in the low incidence of acne among teens from plant eating cultures such as Papua, New Guinea.

Read food labels. Learn how much sugar is poured into commercial food and drink.

Implement healthful, economical, and delicious changes as a family. Give new habits a good six weeks to get established. Try one at a time. Some families use a calendar to chart their progress. Above all, take charge of your family's nutrition.

Children are very curious about their bodies. Engage them in the marvel which they are. I remember spending hours reading from *El Tesoro de la Juventud* the young student's encyclopedia—my favorite section: *El Libro de los Por Qué* (The Book of Why).

It pondered questions like: Why do we need to eat every day? Why do spinach leaves turn yellow the longer they stay in the refrigerator? Why do dry beans double in size when soaked and cooked? What makes a banana ripen as sweet as a date? What gives stools its brown color? Why does an avocado feel slippery when rubbed between the fingers? Why does the lion eat meat while the horse eats plants?

Here are the answers: Because as we burn food for fuel, we need to replenish it. Because plucked from the soil and away from sunlight they stop making green chlorophyl and the orange and yellow carotenes can show themselves. Because they soak up water as they rehydrate. Because as fruits ripen, their carbohydrates break into sweeter simple sugars. Because it is mixed in with bile which is dark green yellow brown in color. Because it is eighty percent fat. Because the lion cannot properly digest plants and the horse cannot properly digest meat.

Olfactory nerve endings within the nose are part of the experience we call taste. Teach children how to tell spices by smell: add chopped dill to a cold salad, a dash of cinnamon to the morning oats, a sprinkle of cumin to chickpeas, a drop of vanilla to a plum. Suffering from a cold or from nasal allergies we have trouble discriminating between some tastes. Pinch your nose and smell or taste for yourself.

Build food literacy. There are countless opportunities to teach children about food and nutrition. Share your questions. For example: What makes peanut a legume and not a nut? How do we keep a knife sharp?

And then share you answers: They are both seeds, but legumes grow in a soft pod while nuts grow in a woody shell. Lightly drag the edge of the knife along the surface of a sharpening stone a few times, keeping a twenty degree angle.

Avoid keeping at home anything that needs to be rationed or limited, like soda, ice cream, cookies, or candy. Reserve these for the occasional party. Focus on providing only nourishing foods. A child will stop eating when she feels satisfied; don't ever force a young child to eat. This is disrespectful of the body's innate wisdom and ruins her satiety sensors. Keep in mind that the stomach is roughly the size of one's fist. Overfilling stretches it to varying degrees of discomfort. Never use food as reward or punishment, your child might pay for this with an eating disorder. Children who are eating enough calories have energy to play and study; your job is to make sure those calories are nutritious and not from sweets and junk food.

Ensure that children grow up with cooking skills. Feed their curiosity. Encourage them to be nature students. A child who has something interesting to say about bok choy, quinoa, kabocha pumpkin, or lentils, grows up a more discriminating consumer than the child who only insists on having burgers, nuggets, and pizza. A child who brings a daikon (large white radish the shape of a carrot) to "show and tell" will be surrounded by curious classmates.

When our son was young he had many visiting friends. Some were happy to dine on rice and beans with us, while others discreetly would wait to get home to their favorite meal of macaroni and cheese. Our tomato pie was declined unless it had cheese. A narrow food repertoire not only limits a child's gustatory experiences, it sets him up for imbalances in nutrition.

The way schools promote poor nutrition should outrage any adult, but especially parents and teachers. It frustrates many cafeteria personnel too. The situation is complicated by subsidies, hired food services, and sports dedicated money. The answer is not to bring in more fast food choices, but to have fewer choices that are more nutritious. Find out about your local school and get involved in any way you can. Help schools get out of the fast-food trap.

Imagine a health curriculum teaching children to cook lentils and Brussels sprouts, instead of brownies or cheese pasta. Imagine children celebrating with pomegranates instead of cupcakes (they are both messy, so there is no excuse). Imagine food laboratories where children get to grow, touch, smell, and taste real ingredients. Challenge schools to teach food literacy.

Check out the nationwide curriculum *Food is Elementary* by Antonia Demas, PhD, and be inspired. www.foodsstudiesintitute.org.

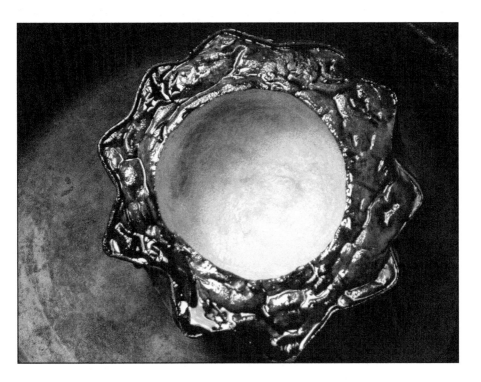

Baked acorn squash—a visual treat. Taking into account the wavy exterior, cut in half and scoop out the seeds. Place cut side down in a dry ovenproof glass pan. Bake for almost one hour at 400° until the aroma of its caramelized sugars permeates the kitchen. Makes me wish I could add a scratch and sniff page to the book.

6

Social Ripples

*H*ealthier food choices might unsettle people around you or bring unexamined feelings to the surface. People unsure of their own eating habits might say you are being extreme for denying yourself a treat. Some fear you won't be going out to eat with them anymore. Others will pronounce that you are just going through a phase. Take these opportunities to clarify your own intentions for eating healthier foods. Practice expressing them in few words. You might irritate some people, but you will inspire a handful and even make new friends. Let people express their views. Don't embarrass them on purpose. There is no need to be confrontational.

Perhaps the following responses could spark some of our own:

Q. Why are you making these changes?

A. They seem to be helping me.

Q. Where do you get your protein?

A. I recycle my own, get the rest from plants.

Q. Aren't you afraid you will get weak?

A. I feel strong and not bogged down.

Q. You need to drink milk.

A. Cows, horses, and many humans, don't drink any.

Q. I don't think I could do it.

A. This lifestyle may not be for everyone.

Part II

Nourishment

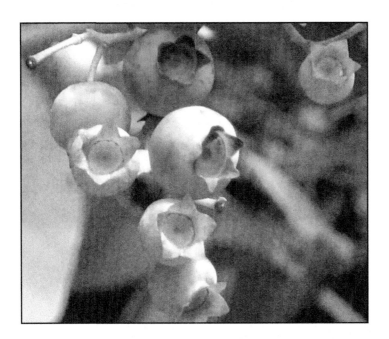

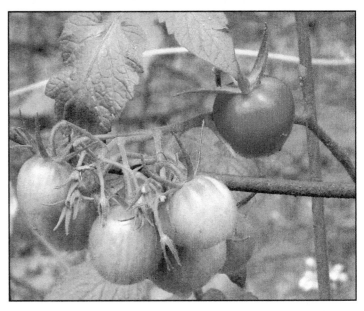

Fruits are the offspring of a flowering plant. The seeds which grow protected inside the fruit are capable of developing a whole new plant if they fall on favorable ground. Blueberries, tomatoes, mangoes, pumpkins, grapes, and okra, are all fruits.

7

The Typical American Diet

*M*any Americans have adopted a parade of party foods as every day fare: pizza, chicken nuggets, salty snacks, soda, sweets, and ice cream to name a few. The typical kitchen is stocked with boxed cereals, bread, chicken parts and other meats, boxed entrées, cold cuts and cheese, assorted bags of leafy greens, yogurt, energy bars, juice and milk by the gallon, and cases of vitaminized water. Compared to people in other developed countries Americans eat fewer home cooked meals citing lack of time and energy. Many are under the impression that home cooking is more expensive than fast food. Riding this wave for over fifty years has visibly promoted disease instead of health. Let's examine these concerns.

TIME: Of course cooking takes time, but insisting that cooking takes too much time bypasses logic. Steel cut oats cook uncovered and without supervision in twenty minutes. Rolled oats are ready in five. A pot of rice cooks alongside a pot of beans, just set the timer. Buy ingredients for two simple recipes (look some up in this book) and in two hours you will have enough food to pack lunch or reheat for the week. The way you chose to spend each day is the way you spend your life. Do what is important to you.

EFFORT: Living solo? Invite friends and turn cooking into a social event. Prepare enough and everyone takes home another meal. Within the family let others help. Whether shopping, chopping, or mixing, there is a job for each person. Ingredients such as onions, peppers, carrots, and some greens, can be chopped in advance and saved in containers, ready for when you need them. You know when you chopped them and that they will stay fresh for two or three more days. Cook in stages. For example, bake whole beets, sweet potatoes, and pumpkins and use them by themselves or in recipes throughout the week.

MONEY: The notion that convenience saves money is a collective delusion. A box of 8 instant packets of oats costs $4; whereas a pound of oats sells for under $2 and will feed one for a month. According to recent statistics, the average American worker shells out more than $20 a week on coffee one cup at a time (a yearly average of $1,000) plus almost $2,000 on take out lunch, thereby lining the pocketbooks of the food industry while emptying her own. (In addition to the instant breakfast and the caffè latte we are getting unwanted extra calories.)

CONVENIENCE: In the 1950s TV tables sprouted across the nation and many families ate breaded entrées like the Swanson frozen dinners out of aluminum trays. Today we unwrap the same lackluster ingredients on the run. We could refashion convenience for the twenty-first century if we cooked once or twice a week and built a nutritious food bank right at home. Visit the recipes in this book and note the ones you could freeze.

EXCESS: Many people used to die of malnutrition, rickets, scurvy, congenital defects, and of infections such as tuberculosis—conditions which plagued our great-grandparents generation before science and technology helped conquer them. How pathetic that we should now die from excess food and over-consumption.

NUTRITION EDUCATION: Thirty-five years ago, *Harrison's Principles of Internal Medicine* offered this guide on nutrition: eat low in fat mostly plants and limit the salt. In one line my medical school text book delivered this crisp and powerful message then left it at that. No more was said on how to deliver this information to our patients or how earnestly we should use this in our practice to protect their health. No mention of the fact that food is powerful non prescription medicine. As a result of this meager nutrition education, physicians have not developed into a credible resource of nutrition information. As for patients, they cannot fully imagine how we could use food to protect health or that nourishing food could arrest and reverse disease. This sorry state in nutrition literacy needs to be addressed with a medical school curriculum that teaches food in medicine.

Periodic testing and scheduled surveillance unaccompanied by meaningful changes in lifestyle and diet make little sense. Too many health professionals subject patients to untold medication side effects for conditions that are reversible. Patients deserve much more from us. Even without health insurance one can adopt a diet that is low in fat mostly plants and limits the salt (like my medical text book suggested). We don't need insurance approval or anyone's permission to do this and we would greatly reduce health care costs.

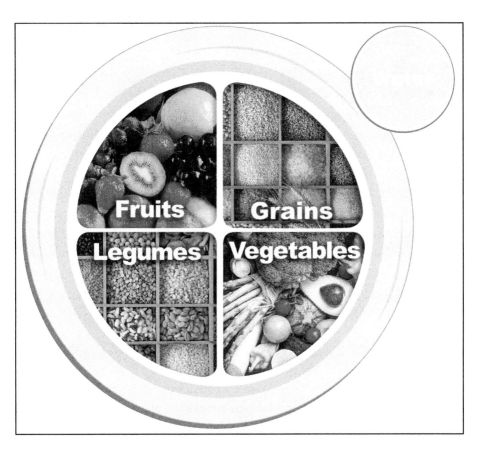

Sustainable Power Plate. Physicians Committee for Responsible Medicine (PCRM) reminds us that unprocessed whole plant foods should make 90% of our diet and recommends this colorful illustration for the 2015 USDA Dietary Guidelines for America.

8

Dietary Guidelines Every Five Years

*I*n a very embarrassing 1967 report, images of skinny children with big bellies were televised into every U.S. household. In the span of one week innocent Americans learned that diseases thought to be the exclusive calamity of third world countries also plagued this land of plenty. The government was alarmed and responded by assigning a Senate committee to investigate the nation's hunger and malnutrition. The group led by George McGovern focused its investigation on lack of food among vulnerable groups and on the gross maldistribution of nutritious food, but was unprepared to discover that diseases of malnutrition were not limited to lack of food. In just a few decades after the World War II a diet of excess fat and sugar had spawned an increasingly overweight population which was dying of cancer, stroke, diabetes, and heart disease—by then already the number one killer. The group issued then what were felt to be clear and much needed nutritional guidelines for consumers:

1. Increase carbohydrate intake to 55-60 percent of calories (by that they meant grains, fruits, and vegetables).
2. Decrease fat intake to no more than 30 percent of calories, with less saturated fat (which meant less meat and dairy).
3. Decrease cholesterol intake to 300 mg per day, (which they stated meant less meat, eggs, and dairy products).
4. Decrease sugar intake to 15 percent of calories, (which meant less pastries, and less processed or refined carbohydrates).
5. Decrease salt intake to 3 g per day.

While the public clearly stood to gain (in nutrition and in health) with this report, the words "decrease" or "eat less" did not sit well with the food in-dustries. They mounted a strong defense / offense retaliation which to this day has not lost steam and sadly none of the committee targets were met. Research teams today are hired to discredit disagreeable data, tout the benefits of their product, and popularize ditties with a scientific ring such as: Milk, it does a body good. In Got milk? even government figures are persuaded (without pay) to wear a white mustache for the dairy campaign—mountains of marketing stand between consumers and the truth.

Despite all hurdles these early reports established a firm link between food and health and with each passing year the recommendations became clearer. A full ten years after the first report the committee did not mince words and issued Dietary Goals for the United States exhorting people to eat more plants and less animals. As expected, tensions mounted again as now the food industry would have to vie not just for a place at the American table, but for the number of servings of their meat, eggs, milk, cheese, sugar, oils, and salt.

The pendulum continues to swing back and forth. However, what began in the late sixties as the innocent investigation into hunger and malnutrition turned into a movement which sought to improve the nation's health on many fronts. A program of foods stamps was established. Important legislation laid the ground for the National School Lunch Act and for the Child Nutrition Act. In an enduring legacy, since 1980 and every five years, the U.S. Department of Health and Human Services (HHS) and the U.S. Department of Agriculture (USDA) jointly publish a continually improving *Dietary Guidelines for Americans*. Having said that and as laudable as this is, it is virtually impossible for these agencies to simultaneously support our health and the health of the food industry or do it consistently. Their conflicting recommendations are symptomatic of the compromising elements tied to subsidies and political favors.

In 1999 the court ruled against the USDA for conflicts of interest and financial ties to various food industries in six of its eleven committee members and for refusing to provide information involving a payment of over $10,000 to one of them.

The 2010 guidelines (the most recent as of this book's publishing date) are summarized in a round plate and a drinking glass, a visual improvement over the former pyramids.

The plate is divided into quadrants labeled: vegetables, grains, fruits, and protein (without naming a source). Since we need only 10% of our calories from protein and every plant especially legumes are an adequate source of this macronutrient, naming a quarter of the plate "protein" is code for meat which for the first time in our history is not considered a food group and won't go without a fight.

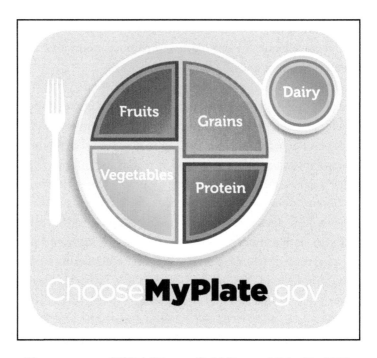

The most recent USDA Dietary Guidelines published in 2010.

For the most part the document is accurate and educational. It confirms that we should eat leafy greens, colorful vegetables, grains, legumes, and fruits, while limiting saturated fats and processed foods. However, it also contains statements promoting dairy, meat, egg, sugar, and oil which contradict the tone of the recommendations. This means that readers without a firm grasp on food literacy are kept deliberately confused while the fight over our food dollars continues. (The Dietary Guidelines could be recommended school reading and would spark interesting discussions among students in class.)

The 2010 guidelines admit that fortified soy beverages count as dairy, affirm that some milk products are not a source of calcium, and correctly state that we should get our calcium from a variety of leafy greens. However, in a blatant advertisement from one of the most powerful food lobbies in the country the glass touching the plate is labeled dairy. The influence of the industry is so strong that for most people this means the milk from cows. Ever wonder how cows, horses, elephants, as well as many people, get all their calcium from plants; that your favorite animal food ate only plants never meat; or that every mammal (including humans) produce milk without drinking milk?

Before each new publication of the guidelines the government solicits reactions from outside its group of experts. At that time health professionals, teachers, and the general public are invited to comment. The complete document *Dietary Guidelines for Americans* is about one hundred pages and is available online to anyone interested in perusing it, but as you might imagine the committee hears mostly from the food industry and those with a single agenda. They desperately need to hear from informed people (like those reading this book) who can separate accurate nutrition information from biased marketing. The dietary guidelines should strike industry advertisement from their recommendations.

It appears that although the Dietary Guidelines are published according to the Center for Nutrition Policy and Promotion by the USDA and HHS, they are caught in a tight spot between serving the public and serving the industry. This is an important fact because in the final analysis their recommendations affect every government food program: Women Infants and Children (WIC): School Lunches; Supplemental Nutrition Assistance Programs (SNAP); Senior Centers; and the Military.

(Current dietary recommendations suggest the following breakdown of calories: 70% carbohydrates and 20% fat with the remaining 10% as protein; with less than 10% of carbohydrates from sugar; and only 2 grams of salt.)

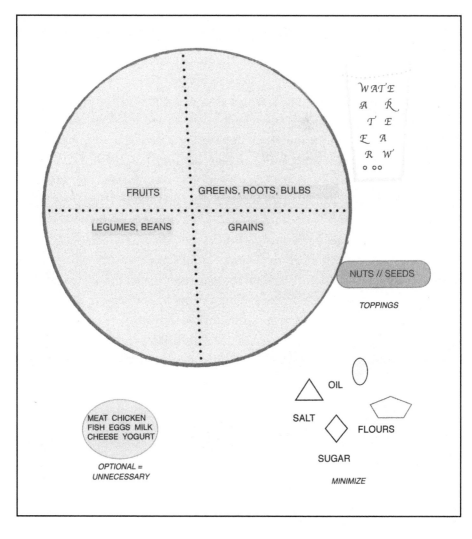

Colorful Plate. Place 90% of your nourishment on the plate using whole or
minimally processed plant foods. Nuts and seeds are nutritious and very calorie
dense—eat only a fistful a day. Animal foods are unnecessary for nourishment,
therefore optional. Factory processed foods are mostly combinations of flour, sugar,
oils, salt, flavorings, and preservatives—keep them in proportion to the rest of your
diet to around 10% of total food for each day. Plants hold a lot of water,
which typically makes up 80-95% of the mass of growing plant
tissues, so on a plant based diet we can eat most of our water.

9

Are We Well Nourished?

*F*rom a point of reference cluttered with misinformation this question may be impossible to answer. Let's look at some common food arguments which are riddled with inaccuracies.

CARBOHYDRATES: Thanks to fad diets and self appointed gurus we are persuaded to avoid carbs, which are in fact our source of energy. What we should avoid are sugars and flours which are the primary ingredients in items such as soft drinks, water ice, ice cream, candy, boxed cereals, bagged snacks, cookies, and pastries. These concentrated carbs deliver too many calories and not much else.

PROTEIN: Although a diet based on plants satisfies our protein needs, many coaches, trainers, and even health professionals insist that we add more protein to the diet usually meaning meat. This idea belongs in the nineteenth century when protein (named proteus for primary) was believed to be the basic unit of life. In truth, protein consists of smaller units called amino acids. These building blocks are shared by every plant and animal on the planet and get rearranged in countless different sequences, which explains how the body can take protein from plants (such as beans, nuts, and rice) and make human protein (such as muscle, skin, and hormones with myriad functions). Children eating enough calories get enough protein. We don't need meat protein to build muscle, we need exercise.

VITAMINS AND MINERALS: Bones naturally make us think calcium and the dairy industry pours billions of dollars to make calcium synonymous with milk. One of their most successful strategies consists of distributing biased educational materials to schools, physicians, and coaches, who in turn disseminate the myth that milk, cheese, and yogurt are essential for strong bones. There is no question that cow's milk is a source of calcium, but its role in a number of conditions such as acne, constipation, and cancers, makes it an ill-advised food for humans of any age.

Calcium makes up seventy percent of the bone; but the remaining thirty percent of our skeleton is a living network of proteins. Weight bearing exercises such as walking and jumping give bones a reason to stay strong and flexible. Along with enough Vitamin D (to retain calcium in the bones) weight bearing protects against osteoporosis. Non weight bearing exercises such as swimming or cycling have cardiovascular and other health benefits, but do not protect against calcium loss. For this reason in the weightless space environment astronauts lose bone mass and need to rebuild it when they return to Earth. Similarly previously bedridden patients must have physical therapy to recover bone loss. Calcium needs of around 1000 milligrams a day, can be met consuming a variety of plant foods (such as collards, cabbage, broccoli, almonds, seaweed, tempeh, and calcium fortified foods). Think of the large animals that walk the planet (elephants, giraffes, horses, cows, orangutans). Where do they get their calcium? Plants! (See Calcium in Foods.)

The Got Milk? dairy ad campaign, which as of 2013 costs twenty-million dollars a year, features public figures with a white mustache spreading unsubstantiated claims that milk helps build muscle and can contribute to weight loss.[1]

REFERENCE:[1] Calcium and Milk: What's Best for Your Bones and Health? Harvard School of Public Health.

SUPPLEMENTS: The powerful supplements industry parallels pharmaceuticals in breadth, scope, and allure. Americans spend 25 to 30 billion dollars a year on their products trying to boost the immune system and stave off disease in spite of scientific evidence that they don't. The immense variety of phytochemicals, vitamins, and antioxidants found in plants, work in concert with each other. This natural condition has yet to be reproduced in powders and pills.

DISSONANCE: What we know and what we practice are often at odds. For example: in spite of consuming too much meat, we still worry we don't have enough protein; and despite limited and unhealthy selections, we still choose fast food for convenience.

Dissonance on a larger scale is even more troubling. For example: the

USDA admits that almost no child eats the recommended amount of fruits and vegetables, yet tolerates a scandalous absence of them in the school cafeteria; in spite of record profits reported by the meat and dairy industries, the government continues to grant them century old subsidies; and while the American Heart Association strongly advises limiting sugar (3 teaspoons for children, 6 for women, and 9 for men) it is poured into almost every processed food in the market.

Back to the question of whether we are well nourished—on the whole we are not. An important goal of this book is to replace misinformation with sound scientific evidence to get us better nourished.

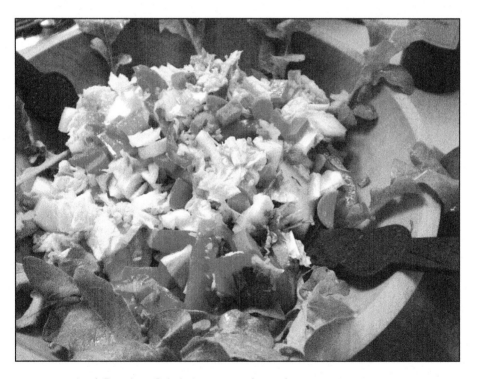

A Rainbow Salad in any one of its infinite permutations
is limited only by the imagination.

10

Macro and Micro Nutrients

*T*his first part of the chapter introduces three macronutrients: carbohydrates which we need in largest amount since they supply most of our energy plus protein and fat, the two compounds which make up our bodies. The second part of the chapter discusses essential micronutrients such as vitamins and minerals which are needed for myriad biochemical reactions in our bodies, but only in small amounts.

The macronutrient, carbohydrate, is our main source of energy used to power the brain and our movements. Once spent the carbohydrates are not available for recycling; we replenish them only by eating again.

The human body is 65% water and any amount we eliminate or evaporate must be replaced. We do this by drinking plain water and eating an abundance of vegetables and fruits, which are over 95% water. Electrolytes (such as sodium and potassium) are lost in vomit and diarrhea and perhaps during a marathon sweating, otherwise we rehydrate perfectly well with plain water.

Apart from water, our bodies are made of approximately 20% protein and 12% fat. The body is constantly disassembling and reconstituting worn down tissue and blood, recycling its own fat and protein for daily repairs. While we use some dietary protein and fat for energy, these nutrients are not the body's preferred fuel, carbohydrate is.

A plant diet with enough calories is adequate to make up for small loses of protein and fat in shed skin, clipped hair and nails, tears, digestive juices, menstruation, ejaculate, and cells dragged out in urine and stools.

We are already made out of protein and fat, so for maintaining the body and making necessary repairs the calorie distribution in plants closely matches human requirements: 70% carbohydrates, 10% protein, and 20% fat. The nutrient distribution in meats is at odds with our human body needs, especially because it provides us no carbohydrate for fuel.

Example: 4 ounces raw or the equivalent of 3 ounces cooked:

Source	Calories	Protein	Carbs	Fat	% Fat Cal
chicken breast	160	28g	0g	7g	40%
lamb	250	30g	0g	14g	50%
salmon, Atlantic	175	76g	0g	11g	55%
steak (beef T-bone)	450	25g	0g	35g	70%

CARBOHYDRATES: Carbohydrate is the human body's choice fuel. It circulates as glucose in levels ranging from 70 to 120 milligrams per deciliter of blood. A small amount of dietary carbohydrate is stored for emergencies as glycogen and the excess is turned to fat. Susceptible individuals who have developed insulin resistance on a diet high in saturated fats have elevated blood sugar which also causes them to have elevated triglycerides—a blood fat. The good news is that a diet of whole foods from various parts of plants (naturally low in saturated fat) together with regular exercise can drop triglycerides within a couple of weeks and turn insulin resistance back to insulin sensitivity.

Carbohydrates are classified as simple (built of one or two sugars) or complex (made of three or more sugars), but outside the laboratory this definition is inconsequential. Whether from a sweet potato or from a chocolate chip, all carbohydrates break down into single sugar molecules and then into glucose. Instead of fretting over simple or complex we should pay attention to how they enter the body. Do we eat them as whole foods such as oats, beets, sweet potatoes, and cabbage, replete with vitamins, minerals, antioxidants, fiber, and phytochemicals; or in breads, cookies, and sweet drinks, stripped from their whole plant benefits?

FIBER IS A CARBOHYDRATE: Cellulose, mucilage, and pectin, are the carbohydrate portions of the plant which humans cannot digest. Insoluble fiber known as roughage, holds on to water, contributes to satiety, prevents the reabsorption of waste, promotes intestinal motility, and like a sponge helps to drag away waste. Soluble or gelatinous fiber helps reduce the risk of chronic illness by slowing the absorption of fats and sugars. Once considered a passive component of our diet, fiber is a group of carbohydrates which is actually fermented by friendly bacteria in the gut. Broken down into short chain fatty acids they provide valuable nourishment for the colonocytes (cells lining the colon). As these short chain fatty acids get absorbed into the blood they also help regulate glucose, lipids, and the immune system. Each gram of plant fiber generates 2 calories, so thanks to this bacteria-mediated metabolism, fiber could contribute 60 to 80 nourishing calories a day.

A diet rich in plants provides much more than fiber toward overall good health, so rather than fiber supplements we should eat foods high in fiber[5]. Whole plant foods, including grains, fruits, vegetables, and legumes, all rank high in fiber. Peeling vegetables and fruits or removing the hulls of grains reduces fiber content. Consider that while canned vegetables and fruits are high in fiber they have lost healthful nutrients. Other types of processing (such as drying, crushing, and popping) reduce the water-holding capacity of insoluble fiber and make the foods more calorie dense. Avoid juicing methods where the flavorless pulp is collected in a filter since this is a sure way to eliminate fiber. Foods of animal origin (meat, milk, cheese, and eggs) have absolutely no fiber. The hard to chew strands within meat are animal connective tissue with zero fiber of plant kind. On average Americans eat less than 20 grams of fiber a day and should aim for 30 to 40 grams.

REFERENCE: [5] Wong JM, de Souza R, Kendall CW, Emam A, Jenkins DJ: *J Clin Gatroenterol.* 2006 Mar;40(3):235-43. Colonic health: fermentation and short chain fatty acids. The emergence of prebiotics and probiotics aimed at improving colonic and systemic health has rekindled interest in short chain fatty acids (SCFAs). Dietary carbohydrates, specifically resistant starches and dietary fiber, are fermented in the gut producing readily absorbed SCFAs (primarily Acetate, Propionate, and Butyrate). This phenomenon depends on the amounts and species of microflora present in the colon, the food source, and gut transit time. Butyrate has been studied for its major role in nourishing the colon mucosa and in the prevention of cancer of the colon. Acetate (the principal SCFA in the colon) after absorption has been shown to increase cholesterol synthesis. However, because Propionate (a gluconeogenerator largely taken up by the liver) has been shown to inhibit cholesterol synthesis, substrates that decrease the ratio between acetate and propionate could reduce serum lipids and possibly cardiovascular disease risk. Therefore, a greater increase in SCFA production and delivery of specifically butyrate, to the distal colon may reduce the risk of developing gastrointestinal disorders, cancer, and cardiovascular disease.

REFERENCE: [5] A Schatzkin, T Mouw, Y Park, A Subar, F, Thompson: Dietary fiber and whole-grain consumption in relation to colorectal cancer in the NIH-AARP Diet and Health Study. *Am J Clin Nutr* 2007;85:1353–60.

PROTEIN: Whether from beans, broccoli, or fish, protein is split into amino acids then reassembled to form people specific proteins. Within the body, worn proteins also get taken apart and reassembled. Most proteins are recycled with very small amounts being used for energy. The typical not olympic athlete needs enough carbohydrate for fuel and 10% of her total calories from protein (forty to fifty grams), just like the rest of us. Unless we are unintentionally losing weight from famine, anorexia, cancer, frail elderly, or suffering from another chronic debilitating condition, we don't need extra protein. With the exception perhaps of pregnant and lactating women or someone suffering from a catastrophic illness, such as recovering from a severe burn or crushed tissue injury, we meet our protein needs by simply eating enough food.

Besides consuming more than enough fat,[3] Americans consume more than twice the necessary protein and are ill advised to add protein shakes or amino acid supplements to their diet. Animal protein is associated with the initiation, promotion, and dissemination of some cancers.[4] Excess protein which is not used for energy or to rebuild worn parts ends up metabolized into ammonia compounds, converted to urea, filtered through the kidneys, and excreted in the urine. If we want to build muscle, what we need is exercise.

REFERENCE: [3] Marion Nestle, PhD: *Food Politics.*
REFERENCE: [4] T. Colin Campbell, PhD: *The China Study*. Animal protein is not a superior food. It increases our risk of cancer and many chronic illnesses.

According to the Census Bureau Statistical Abstract of the United States on Health and Nutrition, in the year 2012 the average American ate 200 pounds of animal meat, 250 eggs, and 600 pounds of dairy products. That amounts to a daily average of 0.6 pounds of meat, 0.7 eggs, and 1.7 pounds of dairy. Why still ask if we are getting enough protein?

PROTEIN NEEDS:

4-8 years: 20 g protein
9-13 years: 35 g protein
girls and boys 14-18 years: 45 to 50 g p rotein
women and men 19-70+: 45 to 55 g protein

The beef, chicken, egg, pork, and dairy boards, all market their products by sending free "educational" materials to physicians, nurses, teachers, nutritionists, coaches, trainers, and body builders. Accepting these advertisements without question, many misinformed professionals become walking billboards for the industry. The antidote to this self-serving industry misinformation is food literacy.

Although we can say that early humans worked hard for their food, our knowledge of specific eating habits is sketchy at best. Those who lived near edible plant growth gathered berries, tubers, and seeds, supplementing their calories with the occasional hunted animal. Less vegetation hospitable environments forced humans to go after animals and gather plants as they could. However, much has changed because eventually humans planted crops and later built supermarkets. Today we don't forage or hunt for our calories; we simply grab food that caters to our taste and try to rationalize that we need it. Instead of comparing ourselves with the imagined man of the Paleolithic era we ought to locate ourselves in modern times and look at ourselves in the mirror. We need reasonably smaller portions of mostly simple unprocessed plant foods with the least amount of chemicals.

The cow, the elephant, the deer, and the ape get to their formidable size and strength without drinking milk past their infancy or ever eating steak or chicken. A horse gets all his protein and calcium from oats and hay, supplementing his diet with carrots and apples not with protein shakes. The horsepower (rate at which work is done) originally compared the output of steam engines with the power of draft horses—an animal who gets all his 16,000 daily calories (ten times the average human needs) from plants.

REFERENCE: *The Cambridge World History of Food.* Edited by Kenneth Kiple & Kriemhild Coneè Ornelas.

Humans (young and old) need an average of about fifty grams of protein a day. Would you have guessed that this sampling totals over fifty grams of protein? (The grams of protein appear in parenthesis.)

1 cup cooked oats (6), 1/4 cup quinoa (6), 3 cups of fruit (3) plus
1/2 cup cooked rice (3), 1 cup of beans (12), 2 cups bokchoy (2) plus
1 cup Brussels' sprouts (4), 1 cup pumpkin or sweet potato (2) plus
1 ounce of nuts (6), 1 cup chard (3), 1/4 cup sprouted rye (6) plus
1 cup soy milk (7), and an assortment of leafy greens.

FATS: We need only 20% of our calories from fat. All the fat we need for brain and cell function is found in or made from whole plants (where small amounts of fat exist combined with carbohydrates, protein, vitamins, phytochemicals, antioxidants, minerals, fiber, water, and more). We can extract a whopping 9 calories (units of energy) from every gram of fat compared to 4 calories from one gram of carbohydrate, but fat is harder to burn than to store (it takes only 2.5 calories to store 100 calories of fat). This means that if fat is overrepresented in the diet, the body would rather store the fat and burn the available carbohydrate. Additionally, on a diet rich in processed carbohydrates such as breads, pastries, and sweet drinks, we have more carbohydrate than we need and end up turning it into extra fat. Enough cycles like this one and the result is weight gain.

Trans fats (those partially hydrogenated oils added to many processed foods) behave just like the saturated fats in meat, milk, butter, and cheese. Although they are banned as an ingredient, trans fats traces are allowed in processed foods and if one's diet consists mainly of factory foods they can add up to a significant amount. Trans fats elevate cholesterol, induce insulin resistance, and create persistent systemic inflammation, all of which can lead to diabetes, heart disease, and cancers.

OIL: Isn't olive oil good for us? We cannot turn an unhealthy diet into a healthy one by adding olive oil. (A tablespoon of any oil delivers 14 grams or 120 calories of pure fat.) Unless we are eating a diet mostly of plants and have already eliminated butter and margarine, the benefits of olive oil are lost in the mix. Try to get good oils by using the whole food, for example mashed olives, ground flax seeds, or puréed cashews.

THE FATTY ACIDS: Fats (classified based on the number of double bonds along their molecular chains) are grouped into monounsaturated, polyunsaturated, and saturated. Keep in mind that we need fats in small proportion to our total calories and that the body makes all the fat we need except for two essential fatty acids which we must get from the diet (Omega 6 Linoleic Acid and the Omega 3 Alpha-Linolenic Acid). Like most other nutrients fats in the body act in concert and never alone, so this section will not assign special value to any particular food for containing this or that fat. Having said that, you will benefit from learning the basics about this most misunderstood nutrient group.

MONOUNSATURATED FATTY ACIDS: Besides being made in the body monounsaturated fatty acids (MUFAs) are found in olives, avocados, nuts, seeds, soybean, flax, and dark chocolate.

POLYUNSATURATED FATTY ACIDS: Polyunsaturated fatty acids (PUFAs) include two important lines (omega 6 and omega 3) which work on opposite sides of the same coin—anti-inflammatory as well as pro-inflammatory. Depending on their concentrations and other variables they up-regulate or down-regulate myriad functions supporting our dynamic metabolic balance with reactions such as prostaglandin synthesis, cholesterol synthesis, blood clotting, and the absorption of vitamins. Although their optimal ratio seems to be 4 (omega 6) to 1 (omega 3); the typical American diet favors omega 6 fatty acids in a ratio of 20:1.

This ratio has health implications. For example, high concentrations of the omega 6 Linoleic Acid raise pro thrombotic, pro inflammatory, and pro constrictive derived eicosanoids plus inflammatory prostaglandins like prostacyclins, thromboxanes and leukotrienes, all found at the root of many common diseases like heart disease. Since some foods have their own elevated ratio of omega 6 to omega 3, one can exaggerate the relative intake of omega 6 PUFAs by eating too many pumpkin seeds, pistachios, almonds, tahini (sesame paste used to make hummus), and vegetable oils which sneak into almost every processed food in the market.

The essential and very beneficial omega 3 Alpha-Linolenic Acid is converted into two important omega 3 fats: EPA or eicosapentaenoic acid believed to play a role in the prevention of cardiovascular disease and DHA or docosahexaenoic acid needed for proper brain and nerve development. Beneficial

PUFAs of this family are found in: green leafy vegetables like lettuce, broccoli, kale, spinach and purslane; legumes like mung, kidney, navy, pinto, lima beans, peas and split peas; ground flaxseed, chia, hemp, walnuts, and soybeans; and citrus fruits, melons, and cherries.

Cold-water fish (including salmon, tuna, halibut, and herring) in addition to certain algae are often mentioned as good sources of omega 3 fatty acids. Beware: farmed fish (compared to fish who live in clean wild environments) could have almost three times the fat, twice the amount of omega 6, half the amount of beneficial omega 3, and variable levels of pollutants thereby offsetting their benefits.

REFERENCE: Benatti P, Peluso G, Nicolai R, Calvani M: Polyunsaturated fatty acids: biochemical, nutritional and epigenetic properties. *J Am Coll Nutr.* 2004 Aug;23(4):281-302. Abstract: "Dietary polyunsaturated fatty acids (PUFA) impact health through diverse physiological processes, such as the regulation of plasma lipid levels, cardiovascular and immune function, insulin action, neuronal development, and visual function. Ingestion of PUFAs will lead to their distribution into virtually every cell in the body with effects on membrane composition and function, eicosanoid synthesis, cellular signaling, and regulation of gene expression." In other words, dietary PUFAs affect the expression of disease genes.

SATURATED FAT: On top of the saturated fat that we make in our bodies, the average U.S. resident consumes 14 kilos (33 pounds) of cheese plus an additional 120 kilos (265 pounds) of beef, chicken, turkey, fish, shrimp, lobster, crabs, or cured meats each year—the equivalent of three quarters of a pound per day. Between a third and a half of all this dietary fat is saturated, raising blood cholesterol and causing insulin resistance. Saturated fat is mainly found in animal products, but in addition the food industry is allowed to use trace amounts of hydrogenated vegetable oils or trans fats, which behave like saturated fats. If your diet includes processed foods your trans fat consumption could add up.

CHOLESTEROL: Cholesterol is an integral part of the outer membrane of each of our cells and is used to make vitamin D and sex hormones. However, humans, just like apes, cows, and horses, make all the cholesterol they need using plant fats.

Increased saturated fat from a diet of meat and cheese fuels the making of cholesterol. In turn, elevated cholesterol, which is among the criteria used to measure the risk of heart disease, ends up gobbled by macrophages and in the walls of arteries compromising their elasticity. In its infinite wisdom, the body tries to remove the cholesterol from macrophages or foam cells within the walls of arteries. When this removed cholesterol is returned to the circulation it is filtered by the liver and eliminated in the bile. Persistent excess of cholesterol in the bile promotes the formation of cholesterol gallstones.

A plant based nutrition prevents the formation of foam cells (cholesterol filled macrophages) therefore protects us against heart disease and the formation of gallstones.

TRIGLYCERIDES: Elevated triglycerides increase our risk of heart disease and are made from excess calories especially from refined carbohydrates such as flours and sugars.

ARACHIDONIC ACID (AA): We make this important omega 6 fatty acid using plant Linoleic acid and like similar processes this one is also internally regulated, so that we never make more AA than we need. Nevertheless, by consuming foods of animal origin which already contain arachidonic acid (AA), we betray this protective mechanism. Once in the body there are two paths for metabolizing AA—one anti-inflammatory the other pro-inflammatory, the latter being the path of least resistance. This means that excess dietary arachidonic acid favors the metabolic production of pro inflammatory chemicals and exacerbates conditions like arthritis, asthma, atherosclerosis, thrombosis, and tumor proliferation.

Some common pharmaceutical drugs aim to interrupt the conversion of arachidonic acid into (inflammatory) compounds which make platelets sticky, narrow the airways, or upset brain balance. Examples: Cyclooxygenase or COX inhibitors like Celebrex which treat the pain and inflammation of arthritis; Lipooxygenase or LOX inhibitor drugs like Singulair which are used to treat asthma; or anti-mania medications like lithium, valproate, and carbamazepine used to treat bipolar disorder.

MICRONUTRIENTS: We need many vitamins and minerals, but in very small amounts. Because their functions dovetail and overlap, it is best to consume them as part of whole plants where they exist in endless combinations.

Consider this cautionary tale: results from a very publicized study in Finland (Alpha-Tocopherol Beta-Carotene cancer prevention trial) startled researchers as they discovered that even though foods rich in Beta carotenes, such as sweet potatoes, carrots, cantaloupes, and spinach, protect smokers against the risk of lung cancer, when taken as supplements isolated from the whole plant they behaved unpredictably and increased cancer risk[6]. We should not rely on juicing, herbal products, protein powders, or supplements, what we need is an abundant variety of plants in our diets.

As part of the Virtual Kitchen Tour we could also take a look at the stash of vitamins and supplements on our shelves. Keep only those that have been prescribed for a particular reason by a health professional and reevaluate them often. There is no evidence that the indiscriminate use of vitamins and supplements (except for Vitamin B_{12} and perhaps Vitamin D) serves any salutary purpose.

REFERENCE: [6] The Effect of Vitamin E and Beta Carotene on the Incidence of Lung Cancer and Other Cancers in Male Smokers. N Engl J Med. 1994;330(15):1029-1035 Alpha-Tocopherol Beta-Carotene (ATBC) cancer prevention trial.

BETA CAROTENES: Carotenes abound in dark green and orange foods, such as carrots, pumpkins, squash, sweet potatoes, mangos, spinach, kale, and turnip greens. Carotenes are powerful anti oxidants in their own right and are the precursors of vitamin A.

VITAMIN A: Plants do not make Vitamin A. The enzyme Beta, beta-carotene 15,15'-monooxygenase present in our gut, is responsible for splitting a molecule of plant Beta carotene into two molecules of vitamin A. This internally regulated mechanism makes all the Vitamin A we need and since this vitamin is fat soluble and gets stored in our fatty tissues, it is rare to ever develop a deficiency. Having said this, Americans consume twice the recommended amount of already made Vitamin A from foods like meat, eggs, shrimp, cheese, and fortified cereals. Excess Vitamin A has health consequences: it interferes with Vitamin D which keeps calcium in the bone, inhibits the work of osteoblasts (bone building cells), and at the same time stimulates osteoclasts (the cells which break down bone). Therefore too much Vitamin A whether from the diet or from supplements can lead to bone loss and increased risk of hip fractures. Furthermore, Vitamin A is excreted in breast milk and its benefits or dangers to the infant when present in large amounts are unknown.

IRON (Fe): Absorption of this mineral is strictly regulated by the body: the less iron we have stored the more we absorb and the higher our bone marrow stores the less we absorb. In spite of the widespread use of milk, calcium supplements, and remedies for acid reflux, all of which interfere with iron's balanced absorption, only 3% of the US population is iron deficient. Unwarranted use of iron supplements could mask hidden blood loss or malabsorption. Indiscriminate use of iron supplements could also put unsuspecting hemochromatosis patients at risk. In hemochromatosis (one of the most common genetic conditions in the USA affecting 0.5% of the population) the person absorbs unchecked amounts of iron causing dangerous levels to be stored in liver, heart, and pancreas. The best way to keep normal iron stores is by consuming foods high in iron (such as beans, tofu, spinach, raisins, and fortified grains) as part of a healthy diet. Check with a health care professional during periods of increased demands, such as childhood or pregnancy when the typical American diet may prove insufficient in iron.

CALCIUM (Ca): The daily amount of dietary calcium necessary[7] to maintain a neutral calcium balance (where the amount lost in the urine equals the amount absorbed in the gut) is not difficult to achieve on a plant based diet. Keep in mind that after a high protein meal (for example of meat or cheese), the ensuing blood acidity is buffered by pulling calcium from the bones, causing a negative calcium balance where the amount lost is greater than the amount absorbed. People living in developed countries where the intake of meat and milk is highest are constantly chasing their calcium losses. In other words the western diet promotes osteoporosis through calcium loss.

REFERENCE: [7] USDA Agricultural Research Service Grand Forks Human Nutrition Research Center Published in the Journal of Clinical Nutrition 2008

We owe bone strength to healthy elastic living tissue[8] since bones that are simply calcium dense may be brittle. According to the US Preventive Services Task Force (a panel of health care experts that evaluates clinical preventive services and the latest scientific evidence on them), the way to avert risk of fracture as we age is with: weight-bearing exercise, improved strength and balance, vitamin D, and adequate intake of dietary calcium (supplemented if necessary). As in most animals and many humans, a diet which includes enough plants supplies enough calcium.

REFERENCE: [8] *Bulletin of the World Health Organization*: vol.81 no.11 Genebra Nov. 2003 Print ISSN 0042-9686; Exercise interventions: defusing the world's osteoporosis time bomb. In this important report The World Health Organization emphasizes "Physical activity is vital for maintaining healthy bones throughout life and is an important factor in preventing osteoporosis, reducing falls, and decreasing the risk of hip fractures. The alarming increase in prevalence of osteoporosis apparently expresses a pressing need for a more active lifestyle among people of all ages. The key benefits of regular physical activity have been well proven — the challenge to policy-makers and health professionals is to determine how to promote it among the general population. National and local policies should be developed and campaigns devised to improve public awareness of the need for active living, accompanied by well-conceived programmes to make physical activity easier and more rewarding. The best way we can help defuse the world's osteoporosis time bomb and prevent unnecessary suffering and mounting health care costs is by taking action now." Does your neighborhood promote strong bones with sidewalks and foot paths for all age groups?

Published research has concluded that a daily calcium intake of around 1000 milligrams is sufficient for the average adult. However, the Dairy Council continues to frighten us with dissolving bones. This with support from the medical industry, aggressive lobbying, and protected status from the USDA, forcing the perennial anxious question, am I getting enough calcium? Just like horse, elephant, cow, deer, hippopotamus, ape, and many humans, we get this amount of calcium by eating an abundance of plants. Weight bearing exercise together with enough Vitamin D and calcium insure the health and strength of our bones. Food literacy regarding sources of calcium and foods that steal it from our bones can dispel myths fuel by greed.

VITAMIN D: This fat soluble vitamin (better called a hormone for technical reasons) is made on sun exposed skin. Full body exposure to noon sun for 30 minutes releases 20,000 units of Vitamin D into the bloodstream and we need around 1,000 international units of Vitamin D a day, so a fair skin person makes enough Vitamin D after exposing face, neck, and arms to the sun for 15 minutes. However, current rampant low levels of Vitamin D are associated not only with poor bone health but also cardiovascular diseases, high serum lipid concentrations, inflammation, glucose metabolism disorders, weight gain, infectious diseases, multiple sclerosis, mood disorders, declining cognitive function, impaired physical functioning, and all-cause mortality. Why are so many conditions associated with low Vitamin D? This alone should be a red flag and perhaps point to some pervasive environmental condition, especially since high levels of the vitamin have not correlated with lower incidence of disease and because supplementing with the vitamin has had no effect on any of the above conditions. What these findings suggest is that low levels of Vitamin D are a _marker_ of disease. In fact, believing that our low levels of Vitamin D are the cause of chronic illness rather than the result might be distracting us from addressing our glaring diet and lifestyle imbalances.

VITAMIN B_{12}:The successful laboratory manufacture of vitamin B_{12} remains one of the great feats of the twentieth century. Animals do not make vitamin B_{12}. Plants do not make vitamin B_{12}. All the naturally occurring B_{12} is made by several strains of bacteria living in the hollows of our guts. Unfortunately, these bacteria which live in the intestinal lumen of animals work distal (further down the gut) to where the vitamin can be absorbed, therefore animals make this essential vitamin in an act of generosity, for others. In the natural world, (except for cows and other ruminants who regurgitate and chew their cud) animals secure B_{12} by eating plants contaminated with feces—the largest reservoir of naturally occurring vitamin B_{12} on the planet.

Most of the B_{12} that escapes the liver ends up in the bile and in the gut, from where it gets reabsorbed and channeled back to the liver insuring that only tiny amounts of B_{12} get lost in the stools. According to this and even without daily ingestion of B_{12} it may take several years before we deplete our liver reserve. If you are curious to know the extent of your B_{12} stores the only way to find out is not from a blood test but from a liver biopsy (only of academic interest), so take your vitamin. People can get small amounts from milk and meat but this vitamin is stored mostly in the animal liver (it is the only water soluble vitamin stored in the liver), so it is prudent to secure it from a supplement. The widely available and typical non-cyanocobalamin form of vitamin B_{12} in supplemental form is methylcobalamin and doses of 1000 micrograms a day are sufficient for most normal adults. (Note that cyanocobalamine doses are very different and in the range of 2.4 micrograms daily.)

NITRIC OXIDE (NO): This gas (not the nitrous oxide (N_2O) or laughing gas that you breathe at the dentist's) is made right within the blood vessels imparting them elasticity. Not having enough nitric oxide results in stiff arteries which are associated with high blood pressure and heart disease. Unable to dilate, stiff arteries deliver insufficient blood to oxygenate our tissues be it the heart or the legs especially during exercise resulting in symptoms like chest pain (angina) and calf pain (intermittent claudication).

The first step in the production of this gas involves chewing and swallowing nitrate rich plant foods such as any kind of vegetable, grain, or fruit. Once absorbed the circulating nitrates are picked up by the salivary glands who secrete them back into the mouth. Specialized bacteria turn nitrates into nitrites and in this new form they are again swallowed and absorbed. Back in circulation, the final step takes place in the walls of arteries where the enzyme nitric oxide synthase converts nitrites into the biologically active nitric oxide gas (NO) insuring that arteries remain elastic. (Larsen et al., 2010)

In the U.S. alone, almost 10% of men have erectile dysfunction due to stiff arteries. During sexual excitation stiff arteries cannot dilate to collapse the accompanying veins which is how blood gets trapped in the shaft, therefore the penis remains flaccid. Many men want to treat their erectile dysfunction with a pill, but combining drugs like sildenafil (Viagra) or tadalafil (Cialis) with heart medicines (such as nitroglycerin or amyl nitrite) could end tragically. Because all of these drugs are nitric oxide donors and impart temporary elasticity to the arteries, they are potent vasodilators. Profound dilatation of the arteries while the pill is in effect can cause a severe enough drop in blood pressure to compromise oxygen flow to the eye, heart, or brain causing blindness, heart attack, or stroke.

It is however remarkable that within days of replacing processed and animal foods with plant foods, the resulting increase in nitric oxide helps reverse hardening of arteries, high blood pressure, and erectile dysfunction.[9]

REFERENCE: [9] Hord NG, Tang Y, Bryan NS: Food sources of nitrates and nitrites: the physiologic context for potential health benefits. *Am J Clin Nutr* 2009;90:1 1-10. The provision of nitrates and nitrites from vegetables and fruit may contribute to the blood pressure lowering effects of the Dietary Approaches to Stop Hypertension or DASH diet.

Nitrates and nitrites were first found in cured meats and the initial research focused on the increased production of certain types of nitrosamine carcinogens which was especially true when animal products with added vitamin C like bacon were cooked at high temperatures. Indeed the increase in these carcinogens was 140 fold, but the data became confusing when we learned that nitrates and nitrites are even more plentiful in the plant world, moreover since in vegetables and fruits these chemicals reduce the risk of harmful carcinogenic compounds. Subsequently rather than blaming the nitrates, the focus has shifted to the health hazards of meat.[10, 11, 12]

REFERENCES:
[10] JO Lundberg: Biology of nitrogen oxides in the gastrointestinal tract. *Gut.* 2012;0:2012 gutjnl-2011-301649v1.
[11] RU Hernández-Ramírez: *Int J Cancer.* 2009;125(6):1424-30
[12] Kuhnle GG, Bingham SA: Dietary meat, endogenous nitrosation and colorectal cancer. *Biochem Soc Trans.* 2007 Nov;35(Pt 5):1355-7.

Gastric cancer risks are observed higher among individuals with low intake of some beneficial plant chemicals such as polyphenols and high intake of animal-derived nitrate or nitrite, when compared to high intake of the polyphenols and low intake of animal nitrate or nitrite respectively. Regarding intestinal and other diffuse types of gastric cancer, polyphenol type antioxidants in pears, mangos, carrots, squash, and legumes, show a protective effect by inhibiting the formation of cancer promoting amines.

PHYTO-CHEMICALS (chemicals that occur naturally in plants): Studies continue to show that when isolated from their original source or indeed from each other many phytochemicals act unpredictably. As of today, we cannot bypass excellent nutrition by loading up on capsules and powders. Money spent on vitamins and supplements is better spent eating more whole plant foods such as oats, blueberries, kale, broccoli, rice, beans, and the like. There are no documented benefits for routinely taking any supplement other than Vitamin B$_{12}$ in doses of 500 to 1000 micrograms of methylcobalamine daily.

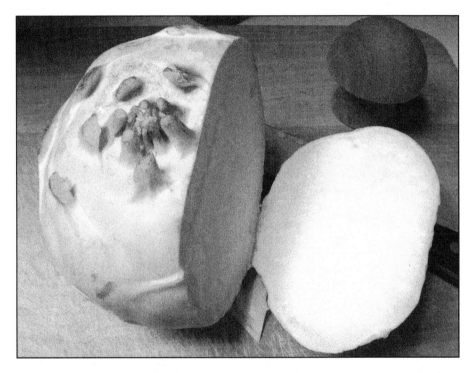

Kohlrabi. Raw slices of this swollen stem, also from the Brassica family, make crunchy chips for humus, dips, and salsa.

11

Using the Nutrition Facts Label

$\mathscr{W}$hole plant foods such as oats, apples, beans, corn, or broccoli, are not required to have a nutrition facts label, what we see is what we get. The nutrient balance of whole plant foods is comparable and easy to understand: mostly energy giving carbohydrate, a little protein, and with few exceptions very little fat. To top it all, these nutrients are found in the proportion that humans need for health and nutrition. The only plants with high fat content are soy beans, peanuts, seeds, nuts including coconut, and avocados.

Processed foods are a different story, which is why the Food and Drug Administration (FDA) requires all manufactured products to have an explicit nutrition facts label that must include:

Serving Size
Servings Per Container
Calories Per Serving
Grams Of Carbohydrate, Protein, Fat, and Fiber
Vitamins
Sodium, Calcium, and Other Minerals
Plus a Full List of Ingredients

Review of terms:

Kilograms, grams, milligrams, and dry ounces express mass
(interchangeable with weight).
Gallons, liters, milliliters, cups, teaspoons, tablespoons, and fluid ounces
    measure volume.
Calories represent units of energy.

It is hard to imagine that before the Nutrition Facts Label became law in 1973 we had no way of knowing what was in Cheese Whiz, Spam, hot dogs, Cool Whip, Ritz Crackers, Tasty Cakes, bologna, or Wonder Bread. Today's products try to fly under our sophisticated radar with name modifiers, for example: organic cheese, lean ground beef, fat free cookie, sugar free ice cream, whole wheat muffin, nut spread, underscoring the importance of studying the label. Learn to spot patterns. For example, manufacturers of boxed cereal manipulate portion size to keep an attractive number of calories per serving plus they use different names for added sugars, to keep you from being alarmed.

NUTRIENTS: All foods share three main nutrients (carbohydrates, protein, and fat), which when metabolized generate calories. Calories are the units of energy we get from each gram of the specific nutrient (each gram of protein or carbohydrate generates 4 calories and each gram of fat 9 calories).

PRACTICE EXERCISE:

Have paper and pencil in hand, so you can do the math as we go along.
Look at the nutrition information of some items in your own kitchen (cans, bags, boxes, and such).
Using the above formula, a 15 ounce can of beans would break down as follows:
3.5 servings each of 0.5 cup and 100 calories
18 grams of carbohydrate x 4 = 72 calories,
7 grams of protein x 4 = 28 calories,
0 grams of fat x 9 = 0 calories

When we consider the calorie rendering nutrients, we need 70% of our calories from carbohydrates, to supply us with daily energy.

According to the Institute of Medicine we need 0.8 grams of protein per kilogram of body weight or 10% of the daily calories[13]. For someone weighing 60 kilos or 132 pounds this means 48 grams of protein. Our concern for protein is overdramatized—with Americans consuming more than double that amount. If we are eating a variety of foods (not just junk and sweets) and if we are not unintentionally losing weight, we are getting enough protein! This fact cannot be stressed enough.

REFERENCE: [13] Institute of Medicine: Dietary Reference Intakes for Energy, Carbohydrate, Fiber, Fat, Fatty Acids, Cholesterol, Protein, and Amino Acids Released: September 5, 2002

Our fat requirements amount to no more than 20% of our total calories, even though the typical American diet derives over 50% of the total calories from fat. Mindful choices throughout the day could easily keep us within a healthful range. With zero fat, our beans leave us enough leeway.

Sodium (Na) plays an essential role, such as in transporting chemicals across the cell membrane. However, too much sodium promotes stiffening of the arteries and is toxic to our tissues. We should not exceed 1500-2000 milligrams of sodium in a day. (The amount we need is close to the number of calories we need, so keeping the milligrams of sodium close to the calories in a serving we can easily stay on target.) Back to our beans, since the sodium for each 100 calorie serving is 140 milligrams, we probably don't need to add more salt during cooking. Each quarter teaspoon of salt (sodium chloride or NaCl) has 600 milligrams of sodium. If a food tastes saltier to you than tears or blood it has too much salt.

INGREDIENTS: Printed on the product label the ingredients appear in descending order of weight, so our can of fully cooked rehydrated beans should list water first then beans and salt last. Following this convention a can of stewed tomatoes should list tomatoes at the top; and a jar of jam should list fruit before sugar.

Regarding flour, when before grinding the grain has been stripped of its bran and germ you will see it listed as rice flour, whole wheat flour, or quinoa flour. However, if the whole grain was used the label would proudly advertise whole grain flour.

As a rule, look for items with an aggregate of sugars no higher than third down the list of ingredients. Keep in mind that if the product uses different sugars, each one contributes small enough quantities to keep sugar from being listed at the top, even though the product is heavily sugared.

Colorings, additives, and preservatives are not nutrients, yet liver and kidneys are burdened with filtering them out of our system to be eliminated in bile or urine.

PRODUCT ADVERTISEMENT: Claims printed outside of the Nutrition Facts Label are not subject to strict regulations. Read the labels on your children's favorite drinks and fruity snacks. Don't forget bagged treats, cookies, granola bars, frozen meals, pasta sauce, and peanut butter. Scan them for portion size, servings in the container, calories from fat, milligrams of sodium, and added sugars. Check the fine print, it may be hard to read for a reason. This quick assessment helps you decide if you want to bring the product into your home or even have it as part of your carry-on diet.

Manufacturers are aware of our latest craze and lure us with slogans. For example: fat free, carb free, gluten free, cholesterol free, anti-aging, rich in anti-oxidants, heart healthy, gut friendly, plus twisted color coded ribbons to support this or that cause, and the list goes on. These phrases appeal to our current values or beliefs. Read the label before buying.

ALCOHOL: Alcoholic drinks are in a category of their own. When in 1935 Congress passed the Federal Alcohol Administration Act, it recognized a tax potential and did not delegate the regulation of alcoholic beverages to the Food and Drug Administration (FDA), instead it assigned the role to the Treasury's Alcohol and Tobacco Tax and Trade Bureau (TTB). To date, beer and wine are not required to have a nutrition label.

Q. If calories are calories no matter the source, why couldn't we satisfy our needs with chips and similar snacks? By now you are probably able to answer this question yourself.

A. We should not satisfy our needs with chips and similar snacks because they lack the variety of micronutrients embedded in whole plants plus they lack fiber to hold water, so we don't feel full before regretting that we've had too much.

PRACTICE EXERCISE, this time using a typical 8 ounce bag of
   potato chips:
The suggested serving size is one ounce or 15 chips: 160 calories.
One serving has 10 grams of fat which multiplied times 9 is 90 calories
   from fat.
Calories from fat divided by 160 equals 56% fat per serving; a lot more
   than our upper limit of 20%.
Sodium is listed as 170 mg per serving, only slightly higher than the 160
   calories per serving, but do we eat only one ounce?
The entire 8 ounce bag holds 1280 calories, 720 calories from fat (still
   56%), and 1360 milligrams of sodium.
Enough to make one sick all day.

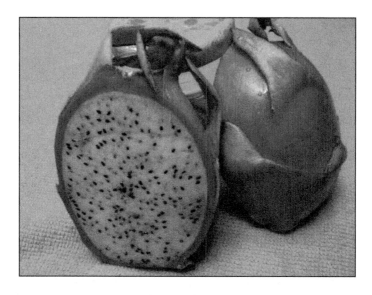

Dragon fruit—beautiful inside and out! This bland watery fruit appears for a short season and has tiny seeds that crunch gently in your mouth. Try it at least once or use it as a model for your art whether watercolors, pastels, or polymer clay.

12

Food Literacy

*E*arly hunter-gatherers enjoyed an occasional animal catch, but extracted most needed nutrients from plants (fruits, roots, leaves, grains, nuts, seeds). Today we gather our edibles on a quick visit to the supermarket and our spear is a fork. We are so dependent on processed (factory) foods that we are missing out on nutritious plants specimens such as kale, kohlrabi, and napa cabbage to name a few.

WHOLE FOODS: A savvy consumer armed with an in depth knowledge of whole foods can buy nourishing ingredients with confidence making every penny count. The delectable flavors in plants are infinite. Ripe fruits are juicy and sweet; freshly picked corn needs no cooking; sugar snap peas are just that; nuts are satisfyingly fatty; oatmeal is gooey comfort; jicama a crunchy crisp. Tickle your senses. Treat your throat to the grit of a pear, cry with onion volatiles, have a pepper sneeze, close your eyes and listen to popping corn. Delight in a rainbow of beets, persimmons, and sprouts. Combine foods and create original new dishes.

For example, during a recent cooking workshop, we chewed on a carrot while commenting on how sweet it was. Then took a pinch of sugar and allowed it to dissolve in our mouths. A few minutes later we tried to eat the rest of the carrots. The facial expressions were priceless, completely baffled. This was the same carrot that a few minutes ago was so sweet? Highjacked by the lump of sugar, our taste buds were unavailable to the sweetness of the carrot. You can see how many children on juice, cereal, or candy, predictably say I don't like broccoli, carrots, or green beans. The good news is that in a couple of days we can lose the taste for excess sugar and acquire a sensibility for the natural flavors in whole food. Plants offer sweetness if only we stopped bulldozing our taste buds with factory drinks and snacks. Try it.

Food factories churn out highly processed and calorie dense foods which have a significant role in today's overweight, obesity, and chronic disease epidemic. They play into our hardwired taste for sugar, fat, and salt. An often overlooked fact is that many times these foods medicate boredom, anxiety, depression, and stress.

SUGAR (sucrose): Sugar is not a whole food and carries none of the benefits of the mother plant from where it was extracted. However, our cells cannot tell if the glucose came from a whole food or from syrup, from an apple or from an apple pie. Once inside our bodies this seductive ingredient turns one hundred percent into glucose.

In 2003 a guide published by the United Nations recommended that manufacturers, cooks, and consumers refrain from adding free sugars to those already present in natural foods, in an effort to limit free sugars to less than 10% of the total energy intake of a healthy diet. The guide was the work of a panel of 30 international experts from the World Health Organization (WHO) and the Food and Agriculture Organization which also maintains that 55% to 75% of our total energy intake should be carbohydrate from whole foods. While all this sounds very official and categorical, according to the 2010 Dietary Guidelines for Americans free sugars still "contribute an average of 16% of the total calories in American diets."

In 2013 the American Heart Association issued a more practical statement. Citing the numerous negative health consequences of excess free sugar, it recommends a top daily limit of: 9 teaspoons of sugar for men, 6 for women, and 3 for children. In other words, most of our sugars should come from the naturally occurring carbohydrate in food not from a bowl. An eight ounce fruit drink has 5 teaspoons of sugar and a twelve ounce can of soda has 10. These 50 to 150 calories could be better consumed in naturally sweet and nutritious whole foods like a cauliflower, a beet, a few dates, or a mango.

We extract and crystalize sugar from sugar cane, but also from beets and dates. It is a travesty that much of our corn is processed into high fructose syrup. All over the world consumers, cooks, and manufacturers add this cheap ingredient to food processing. Our instinct to seek out sugar was lifesaving when it was scarce and part of nature, but we don't live there anymore. As if that was not enough, we also steal honey from bees (around 70 thousand tons in 2011).

Why should we restrict sugar? Whole plants bundle their carbohydrates in fiber, water, antioxidants, vitamins, minerals, protein, and fat, but when we scoop sugar out of a bowl we don't seem to know if we have had enough and we tend to use too much. Apart from the physiologic craving, excess sugar is toxic to us. Prolonged exposure to high concentrations of glucose in the blood increases production of the superoxide anion (O_2^-) a damaging free radical which is implicated in diabetic vascular disease and is currently studied in association with Alzheimer's Disease. Try to get used to less sugar.

Although it appears under many names sugar is sugar in every permutation: sugar, sucrose, glucose, maltose, turbinado, brown sugar, beet sugar, raw sugar, confectioner's, evaporated cane juice, cane crystals, caramel, ethyl maltol, fruit juice concentrate, high fructose corn syrup solids, corn sweetener, treacle, sorghum syrup, maltodextrin, dextrose, dextran, date sugar, high fructose, liquid fructose, molasses, pancake syrup, maple syrup, agave, and honey.

Sugars are unnecessarily added to products such as: peanut butter, spaghetti sauce, boxed cereals, and baked beans. Sugars are the top ingredient in candies, jams, and chocolate bars. Sugar is the only nutrient in soft drinks. Raw agave is a commercially produced syrup from the agave plant with the same 50 calories per tablespoon as sugar. Promoters of agave claim that because it tastes sweeter than sugar we use less of it. Do we?

Sport drinks and other refreshments: Most people down the two serving 16 ounce bottle sport drink in one thirst quenching gulp. Its 100 calories come from six teaspoons of sugar. The same goes for soda, juice, or energy drinks. Eight ounces deliver 120 calories of flavored sugar water. These drinks are sold to children, athletes, and anyone thirsty. Caffeinated sugary drinks appeal to people looking for an energy boost. Store placement, the right container, posing as diet friendly, and suggesting a cool life style, are all marketing ploys. Sugars may satisfy our energy needs, but leave us wanting the nutrients in whole plants plus the health consequences of too much sugar are well documented.

OIL: Oil is not a whole food. Fatty acids are an essential component of our cells plus they facilitate the absorption and transport of fat soluble vitamins throughout the body. (Think of a lubricant that makes things run smoothly by getting into every nook and cranny.)

The best way to obtain fat nutrients is not from oil, but from the whole food: fruits like avocado and olives, whole grains, nuts, and seeds. Because of their high oil content, grains and seeds can turn rancid and develop molds even with proper refrigeration. In the nineteenth century the starchy endosperm of the grain was successfully separated from oily germ and bran and we got white flour. This practice extended the shelf life of baked breads and other grain products overnight since now insects and molds found fewer nutrients to attack. It also meant that each component (the bran, the germ, and the white flour) could be sold separately.

Having a taste for fat was important for the survival of our ancestors (a stroke of genius by the gods), but we have turned this proclivity against us. Separating food into its components simply because we can, we have created concentrations of fat (and sugar) never found in nature. Oil is extracted from fruits like olives and from almost any grain, nut, or seed. No matter whether from olives, corn, rapeseed (canola), sesame, flax, hemp, walnuts, or coconuts, all oils are 100% fat. Able to pour oil out of a bottle, we find ourselves unnecessarily frying rice, noodles, dough, vegetables, chicken, and already oily nuts; mopping oil up with bread; drowning our salads in it. Adding oils to a diet already high in processed and animal foods, we easily consume more than the recommended 20% of our calories from fat.

Nature is self balancing and self regulating, but technology in our greedy hands shows no restraint and we have turned nature's balance upside down. Here are ways to restore it: Buy a small bottle of oil and make it last several months. Don't ever deep fry. Slash the amount of oil in recipes to the minimum that preserves the taste and integrity of the dish. Don't use oil for rice, beans, or soups. Add a tablespoon only to spread the flavors in a salad. Flavor with oil rich foods such as avocado, olives, coconut, cashews, and tahini instead of using simply oil.

The market stays one step ahead of us playing musical chairs as ingredients fall in and out of favor. Regarding fats: butter replaced the once common lard then vegetable shortening and margarine; trans fats fell out of favor and full circle we are back to butter. Overuse of any of these 100% fats is contributing to our overweight and obesity epidemic.

SALT: (NaCl or sodium chloride): Dunes and flats of concentrated salt deposits are found throughout the world. However all plants absorb salts from the soil in which they grow. We should pause before the tendency to pour too much out of a shaker. A quarter teaspoon of salt has 600 milligrams of sodium and enhances many flavors, but excess salt contributes to hypertension by reducing the nitric oxide which keeps arteries elastic.

You could stay within the healthy limit of 1500-2000 mg of sodium a day by choosing foods with matching milligrams of sodium and calories, assuming you need 1500-2000 daily calories. This is easy when buying whole foods since they are naturally low in sodium, but could prove challenging when buying processed foods. For example: a serving of Newman's Own Marinara sauce has 70 calories and 460 milligrams of sodium; Amy's light in sodium Lentil Vegetable soup is 160 calories and 340 mg of sodium. The way to get around this is by adding enough fresh whole ingredients to the marinara or to the soup until the calories match the sodium.

Use the salt shaker at the table rather than during cooking, this way your taste buds get the full salty impact and you are likely to use less. Different salts contain anywhere between 2% and 5% of various other minerals in the mix. Much like in the different sugars these so called impurities add color and flavor, but not necessarily essential nutrients.

Potassium chloride (KCl) sold as a salt substitute is often mixed with ordinary table salt to mask its bitter taste. (The main use of potassium chloride is in fertilizers and lethal injections.) A dash of regular salt (NaCl), a spritz of lemon juice, or commercial combinations of herbs and spices are better choices.

The following ingredients combined with sugar, oils, and salt make up 90% of products on the supermarket shelves.

FLOUR: Flour is not a whole food. Most flours come from refined grains (which means that fiber, germ, and bran were removed). Unless they are labeled whole grain flour, they are more calorie dense than the whole grain. Supermarkets fill the shelves with refined products which combine wheat flour with sugar, oil, butter, milk, eggs, salt, colorings, and preservatives. These products differ only in appearance (take for example: bread, bagels, pancakes, waffles, cakes, muffins, cookies, crackers, pretzels, boxed cereals, frozen tacos, tortillas, and pizzas). See TABLE, Grains.

Grains allowed to sprout may be consumed in this midway form, before becoming a new plant. Sprouted grains are in a dynamic growth phase and their nutrient bioavailability makes them easier to digest for some people. Sprouted grains can be used instead of flour in baking recipes. Simple easy to use sprouting contraptions are sold in Indian stores for ten dollars. The four interlocking stacked pans maintain the right humidity for a couple of days until the seeds germinate. For a satisfying experience start with lentils which sprout a little tail in twenty-four hours.

SPECIALTY MILKS ARE NOT AN ANIMAL PRODUCT: Plant based milks such as soy, almond, rice, hemp, or coconut milks, are plant based refreshments fortified with added calcium. Use them to flavor home cooking; choose based on calories, fat content, sugars, and your intended purpose.

Animal products, such as milk, cheese, meat, and eggs, have been occupying center plate in the American diet and as such play a significant role in the obesity and chronic disease epidemic.

MILK: Insulin like growth factor (IGF-1) is a natural ingredient in milk, but when comsumed by adults is associated with the untimely and unchecked cell multiplication which can lead to some cancers. Milk is excellent food for a fast growing infant, but once weaned we do not need milk (human or from any other animal). All mammals (including us) graduate from mother's milk to the food natural for their species. What we continue to need is calcium, which just like all animals and many humans we can get from plants. See Cancer References.

1% Milk	1% Chocolate Milk
Serving size 1 cup	Serving size 1 cup
Calories 100	Calories 150
Fat 3g or 27% of the calories	Fat 3g
Carbohydrates 12g (mostly lactose)	Carbohydrate 20g (lactose plus sugar)
Protein 8g	Protein 10g

CHEESE: Made from pressed curds of sour milk, cheese contains the protein of the milk. Whether by itself or added to salads, meats, pasta, breads, and oil, this product is ubiquitous in mainstream menus. Cheese is not a healthy food or snack. Consider an occasional sprinkle of nutritional yeast on food for flavor.

14 inch Cheese Pizza	Macaroni and Cheese	Enchilada
Serving Size 1 slice	**Serving size 1 cup**	**Serving size 1**
Calories 300	Calories 500	Calories 350
Fat 10g; 30%	Fat 25g; 40%	Fat 20g; 50%
Carbohydrate 35g	Carbohydrate 40g	Carbohydrate 25g
Protein 10g	Protein 20g	Protein 20g

MEAT: The dietary guidelines of 2010 affirm that meats are not a food group, yet still beholden to the meat lobby the document replaced it with the term protein. Meats lack carbohydrate, which is our main source of energy; they also lack phytochemicals, fiber, protective antioxidants, carotenoids, folate, Vitamin C, Vitamin E, Vitamin K, and many trace minerals essential to health and wellness. Meats (along with cheese) are a source of saturated fat, are disproportionately high in omega 6 fatty acids, and contribute to chronic inflammation. Discounting their appearance, chicken wings, short ribs, and pigs' feet are nutritionally the same:

Pigs' Feet	Chicken Wing	Chicken Breast
Serving Size 1 foot	**Serving size 2 wings**	**Serving Size 1 small**
Calories 200	Calories 200	Calories 240
Fat 14g or 63% of cal	Fat 13g or 58% of cal	Fat 6g or 22% of cal
Carbohydrate 0g	Carbohydrate 0g	Carbohydrate 0g
Protein 19g	Protein 20g	Protein 45g
Vitamin A 0%	Vitamin A 1%	Vitamin A 0%
Vitamin C 0%	Vitamin C 0%	Vitamin C 0%
Calcium 0%	Calcium 0%	Calcium 0%
Fiber 0g	Fiber 0g	Fiber 0g

EGGS: Stocked with about 90 calories (30 from protein and 60 from fat), the egg is an incubator with a pantry. The chick embryo lives inside this protective shell until it comes out twenty-one days later able to care for himself. Each egg has over 250 mg of cholesterol (the recommended upper limit for humans) and lacks any carbohydrate (our main fuel).

FACTORY FARMING

We say we abhor animal confinement, unnatural feed, and antibiotic abuse, which is ironic because these are the same farming practices that satisfy our insatiable appetite for meat and cheese. Catch phrases such as organic, free range, and grass fed, don't describe actual field practices. They are intended to lure the conscientious consumer so he can go on rationalizing a lifestyle dependent on them. Cosmetic modifications such as to the animals' living environment or to the processing plant seem to appease some protesters of factory farming. In the USA ten billion animals are raised and slaughtered annually for food.

From animal handling to processing and packing, factory farms are hazardous environments.[14] One study by the Johns Hopkins School of Public Health found that half of slaughterhouse workers on the killing floor (in constant contact with feces, vomit, and diseased animals) tested positive for campylobacter (a bacteria that can cause diarrhea, stomach cramps, and fever). Investigative journalist Eric Schlosser writes about the meat packing industry as having one of the highest injury rates of any job. Others, like Jennifer Dillard from Georgetown University Law, write about the psychological impact of the killing floor on the slaughterhouse worker. Factory farming is hard on everyone.

REFERENCE:[14] Margo DeMello, PhD. *Animals and Society: An Introduction to Human-Animal Studies.*

Cultural anthropologist Margo DeMello, PhD considers that "one of the reasons that meat is so heavily consumed in American society is because it is produced so cheaply." In addition to a low pay, slaughterhouse work is among the most dangerous in the country. According to the U.S. Department of Labor, workers on the killing floor suffer one of the highest rates of illness or injury within the private sector and the highest in the food manufacturing business. Killing animals as they thrash, kick, or flap, struggling to escape is inherently hazardous.

Factory farming is also hard on the environment. For example, between 2,500 and 10,000 gallons of water are needed to bring one pound of beef to market compared to 25 gallons to produce a pound of potatoes and 50 for a pound of apples. (David Pimentel, PhD, Professor of Ecology and Agricultural Science, Cornell University, Ithaca, New York.) These exaggerated demands on the environment place a moral burden on us as a society especially as we continue to spread our taste throughout the globe.

"In order to maintain his credo, he (modern man) cultivates a remarkable lack of introspection."

—Carl Jung

SUGAR BY ANY OTHER NAME IS STILL SUGAR[15]

This entire section is dedicated to sugars to put one thing in perspective—when we obsess over one ingredient we lose sight of the whole. Our diet must be balanced by an abundance of whole plants, not dominated by one ingredient. A diet is not made healthful by substituting one factory ingredient for another, but by eating a variety of grains, legumes, vegetables, and fruits every day.

Sugar is hidden in almost every processed food, therefore it deserves an expanded section within this chapter on food literacy. Sugar is 100% carbohydrate and there are 4 calories in a gram of carbohydrate, which is important to know because the food label reports sugar in grams.

One tablespoon = three teaspoons.
One teaspoon = 15 calories, 4 grams.
One tablespoon = 45 calories, 12 grams.
The average commercial 12 ounce soda, tea, or juice has 150 calories—all from sugar.
A 16 ounce latte grande has 190 calories—almost all from sugar.
A kid size blueberry water ice has 210 calories—all from sugar.
Half a chocolate bar (2.5 ounces) has 450 calories—most of them from sugar.
Given the above examples, it seems silly to use an artificial sweetener to replace a mere teaspoon of sugar or 15 calories in your regular cup of coffee or tea.

The following list rounds up the number of calories in one tablespoon to the nearest number 0 or 5:

Table sugar is also called sucrose. One tablespoon of granulated table sugar has 45 calories. The U.S. Sugar Association aggressively promotes sugar over artificial substitutes and continuously challenges scientific findings regarding the negative side-effects of sugar consumption.

Agave nectar (more accurately a syrup) is produced from the plant's giant pineapple-like root bulb. The starch of the agave is converted into a fructose-rich syrup in a process similar to that by which corn starch is converted into high fructose corn syrup. Agave nectar consists primarily of two simple sugars: fructose and glucose. One tablespoon has 60 calories. Agave nectar often substitutes sugar or honey in recipes and is added to some breakfast cereals as a binding agent. It is one and a half times sweeter than sugar and since it dissolves quickly can be used as a sweetener for cold drinks such as iced tea.

Honey contains two separate simple sugars fructose and glucose. (Table sugar has the same two sugars, only they are bound together to form a double sugar called sucrose.) One tablespoon of honey is 60 calories.

Molasses sugar is composed of: sucrose, glucose, and fructose. It has 60 calories in each tablespoon.

Maple Syrup is 1% fat, 99% carbohydrate, 0% protein and is 50 calories per 1 tablespoon.

High-Fructose Corn Syrup at a little over 50 calories per tablespoon is artificially achieved, but not significantly different in composition or metabolism from other fructose-glucose sweeteners. Fructose is the simple sugar naturally found in fruits. Manufacturers combine artificial sweeteners with high fructose corn syrup to produce very low-cost drinks which threaten the traditional sugar market.

The craving for high fructose continues to rise in Western societies. Recent studies show that someone who consumes an excessive amount of sugar experiences high extracellular dopamine levels which enhance the desire to consume more sugar. Dopamine is a neurotransmitter that helps regulate reward and pleasure centers in the brain and drops in dopamine relative to acetylcholine (another important chemicals in the brain) cause withdrawal symptoms, similar to those of a person abusing drugs.

Moreover, even moderate levels of fructose in the diet can increase blood glucose and triglycerides levels.

Stevia sweetener is not sugar, therefore it is in a league of its own. Stevia is a plant from the sunflower family widely grown for its sweet leaves and native to subtropical and tropical regions from western North America to South America. It has 300 times the sweetness of sugar, yet its negligible effect on blood glucose makes it attractive to diabetics. As a sweetener and sugar substitute, stevia's taste starts slower and lasts longer than that of sugar. The availability of stevia varies from country to country. For example, in Japan stevia has been available for decades. In the United States it was banned during the early 1990s (unless labeled as a dietary supplement) then it was approved as a food additive in 2008. The disadvantage of using stevia is that it keeps us hooked on excessively sweet tasting foods. It is prudent to use it in very select instances or not at all.

Sugar alcohols [16] retain moisture, add texture to foods, and contain somewhat fewer calories than sugar (about 1.5 to 3 calories per gram of sugar alcohols compared 4 calories per gram of sugar), but they are neither sugar-free nor calorie-free. Although many cakes and pies made with sugar alcohols are marketed to diabetics they do affect blood sugar and when consumed in excess will cause weight gain. Much like fructose (one of the main sugars in fruit and fruit juice), sugar alcohols can have a laxative effect. On the positive side, because sugar alcohols do not cause tooth decay, they are used in sugar-free gums. The following is a list of these sweeteners:

> **Mannitol** occurs naturally in pineapples, olives, asparagus, sweet pota-toes, and carrots and is commercially extracted from seaweed for use in food manufacturing. Mannitol has 50 to 70% of the relative sweetness of sugar, which means we must use more of it to match the sweetness of sugar. Mannitol lingers in the intestines for a long time often causing bloating and diarrhea.

> **Sorbitol** is made from corn syrup and is found naturally in fruits and vegetables. Sorbitol has only 50% of the relative sweetness of sugar, which again means that we need more to effectively sweeten a product. Sorbitol is often an ingredient in sugar-free gums and candies and compared to mannitol tends to cause less diarrhea.

Xylitol (also called "wood sugar") occurs naturally in straw, corncobs, fruit, vegetables, mushrooms, and some grains. Xylitol has the same relative sweetness as sugar. It is used in chewing gums.

Lactitol has about 30 to 40% of sugar's sweetening power but it dissolves and tastes like sugar, so it is often used in sugar-free ice cream, chocolate, candies, pastries, and jams.

Isomalt is 45 to 65% as sweet as sugar and does not break down or lose its sweetness when heated. Because it absorbs little water, it is often used in hard candies, toffee, cough drops and lollipops.

Maltitol is 75% as sweet as sugar. It gives a creamy texture to foods, so it's used in chocolate-flavored desserts and ice cream.

Hydrogenated starch hydrolysates (HSH) are produced from corn and have 40 to 90% the sweetness of sugar. HSH do not crystallize and are used extensively in confections, baked goods, and mouthwashes.

REFERENCE: [15] Michigan sugar education facts.
REFERENCE: [16] Adapted from the Yale New Haven Hospital website.

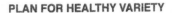

PLAN FOR HEALTHY VARIETY

Fruit: the part of the plant that protects the seeds.

 tomatoes, peppers, pumpkins
mangos, grapes, apples, berries
*avocados

Nuts: seeds that grow inside a woody shell.

almonds, walnuts, pistachios, cashews
other seeds: sesame, sunflower, flax, chia

Grains: seeds of grasses.

 oats, rice, corn, barley, millet, wheat

Legumes or Beans: seeds that grow in pods.

chickpeas, red beans, black beans, lentils, mung beans, moth beans
*peanuts, *soy beans

Leafy Greens, Heads, and Stems:

kale, collards, Swiss Chard,
arugula, cilantro, basil, parsley
Brussels sprouts, cabbage, broccoli, cauliflower
celery, asparagus, kohlrabi

Roots,   Tubers,   Bulbs: parts of the plant that grow underground.

potatoes, sweet potatoes, beets, carrots, radishes, rutabagas, onions, shallots, garlic

Anatomy of a Plant.
Plants store nutrients in various parts of their anatomy—from roots to fruits.

13

Anatomy of Edible Plants

*W*ithin our planet's enormous web of life herbivores eat plants and carnivores eat herbivores. Without plants the herbivores would disappear forcing carnivores to prey on each other and soon vanish themselves. After consuming our stored goods, eventually human food factories would come to a stand still. In the final analysis, plants are our only true source of nourishment.

USING THE ANATOMY OF PLANTS TO SELECT OUR FOOD: Plants are the only makers of carbohydrate on the planet. They store this and many other nutrients in roots, bulbs, stems, leaves, fruits, and seeds. Edible plant parts contain all the protein, fats, carbohydrates, and minerals that we need. Choosing foods according to plant anatomy might encourage us to try something new. From the parts that grow underground, to leafy greens and seeds, all the way to fruits and nuts, sample at least one different food every time you shop. Notice color and shape. Savor. Discover ways to enjoy your new selection (sliced, raw, baked, diced, in a pan dish, or in a succulent soup). Explore the cabbage family (kale, bok choy, napa, Brussels sprouts, kohlrabi, arugula). Soon you will be choosing from a bounty of ever more familiar plants. Visualize the following foods in their growing environment:

UNDERGROUND: Bulbs (onion and garlic) grow alongside rhizomes (of ginger and turmeric). Roots (include beets, carrots, horseradish, and daikon) and tubers (include potatoes and sweet potatoes) are each distinct and full of carbohydrates, carotenes, water, and fiber.

ABOVE GROUND: The thick pale green stem of kohlrabi is crowned by long edible leaves. Asparagus grow tender sticks. Celery is a crisp stringy watery stem. Heads of the calcium rich cabbage family include green, red, and napa. Dozens of the tiny cabbages we call Brussels sprouts grow along a tall sturdy stalk. Leaves from the same cruciferous family such as collards, bok choy, kale, arugula, adorn the ground with undulant greens. Chard, lettuce, and spinach grow straight from the ground. Fragrant herbs grow on spindly stems and include cilantro, parsley, basil, rosemary, tarragon, and bay leaves. Fennel (tastes like licorice) is a compact crunchy bulb with several stalks growing out of it ending in a leafy frond which looks like dill.

NO SAND IN YOUR MEAL: Get rid of the fine dirt which hides in the folds of leafy greens. Remember that they were pulled from the soil. Fill a bowl with cold water. Agitate the leafy greens in the water then lift them out. Feel the bottom of the bowl with your fingers. If it is gritty empty the bowl and refill it with fresh water and rinse again. Repeat until you feel no more sediment at the bottom of the bowl. Don't ruin a dish by skipping this step.

FRUITS: The world's tropical and temperate zones are known for abundant succulent fruit such as tomato, eggplant, okra, pepper, berries, melon, pineapple, zucchini, pumpkin, squash, pear, apple, mango, banana, and avocado. Fruits are babies growing from the fertilized ovaries of flowering plants and trees. Fruits like other edible parts of a plant are rich in carbohydrate, water, fiber, and vitamins. Seeds are usually found inside the fruit with the exception of fruit clusters such as pineapples and strawberries and raspberries which have their seeds on the surface. Seeds under favorable conditions grow into a whole new plant.

SEEDS OF THE HARVEST: We cannot imagine a world without grains. The seeds of grasses such as oats, rice, wheat, corn, barley, quinoa, and millet, grains have been the agricultural cornerstones of civilizations around the globe.

Legumes are seeds that grow inside soft and sometimes edible pods. They are rich in carbohydrate and fat free protein. Beans offer an assortment of tastes and textures and have been named using nearly every letter of the alphabet: adzuki, Anasazi, black beans, black eye peas, cannellini, chickpeas, eye of the goat, favas, lentils, moth, mung, northern, navy, peas, peanuts, pinto, rattlesnake, red, snap, soy, tolosana, wax, and winged.

Nuts are also seeds and most of them grow protected by hard woody shells. Brazil nuts, almonds, cashews, coconuts, hazelnuts, macadamias, pine nuts, pistachios, or walnuts make a fine topping for green or fruity salads. All are very high in fat with chestnuts being the exception.

Herbaceous plants like chia, flax, sesame, fennel, dill, coriander, and hemp are valued for their small oily seeds, laborious to harvest therefore expensive.

Large flavorful seeds such as from sunflowers and pumpkins are enjoyed by many animals including humans. Choose raw seeds without added sugars or oils and dry roast them yourself.

BRASSICA, ALSO KNOWN AS CRUCIFEROUS: Eating from this group of vegetables is said to lower cancer risk. Population studies over the past twenty years find this association most consistently for cancer of the lung, stomach, rectum, and colon; also for cancer of the prostate, endometrium, and ovaries. The most recent data support the hypothesis that eating several cups of brassica each day lowers the risk of breast cancer by as much as 20% to 40%.

Although such statistics are hard to interpret, the cruciferous group of plants has undeniably caught our attention. The sulphoraphanes in these vegetables interact with tumor suppressor gene p53, protecting our cells from cancerous mutations. [17] Chemicals in brassica vegetables stimulate the production of phase II detoxification enzymes in the liver, essential in ridding us of many toxins. See metabolism of free radicals.

REFERENCE: [17] Smith-Warner SA, Willet, WC, Spiegelman D, Hunter D: Brassica Vegetables and Breast Cancer Risk. JAMA 2001;285(23):2975-2977.

Known species of the Brassica family include arugula, bok choy, broccoli, broccoli rabe, Brussels sprouts, cauliflower, Chinese, napa, green or red cabbage, collard greens, daikon and other radishes, kale, kohlrabi, mustard greens, rutabaga, turnips, turnip greens, and watercress. Their different shapes, flavors, textures, and colors, make them the stars in many recipes.

The National Cancer Institute, the National Institutes of Health, and the recent 2010 Dietary Guidelines for Americans, all recommend that we eat four cups of fruit and five cups of vegetables every day. In practical terms, a healthy balanced diet free from junk, animal, and most processed foods, should include two pounds of plants in a great variety of colors every day, especially brassica.

MINIMALLY PROCESSED PLANTS: This category includes fresh, dried, frozen, and canned produce—much of which is found within the center aisles of the supermarket. They are a treasure for the savvy consumer and available year round. The following is only a sampling:

Rice, oats, quinoa, buckwheat, corn, amaranth, wheat, barley, beans, and
lentils.

Dehydrated seaweed, fungi, mushrooms, apricots, dates, and raisins.

Fragrant leaves of thyme, tarragon, basil, oregano, and dill.

Fennel seeds, cloves, and rosemary sprigs.

Ground cinnamon and cinnamon bark sticks; cardamom, coriander,
pepper, turmeric, nutmeg.

Nuts and seeds shelled or not.

Canned beans, tomatoes, pumpkin.

Mixed frozen berries and vegetables retain flavor and nutrition.

Vinegars of various origins, such as apple, rice, date, and grapes (balsamic).

Lime and lemon juice.

Capers, olives, garlic, ginger, and cloves, impart unmistakable taste to many
dishes.

Watch the salt in specialty items like artichokes, palm hearts, and bamboo
shoots.

Beware of dry cranberries, crystalized ginger, or fruit leather, which may
have as much as five teaspoons of sugar per serving.

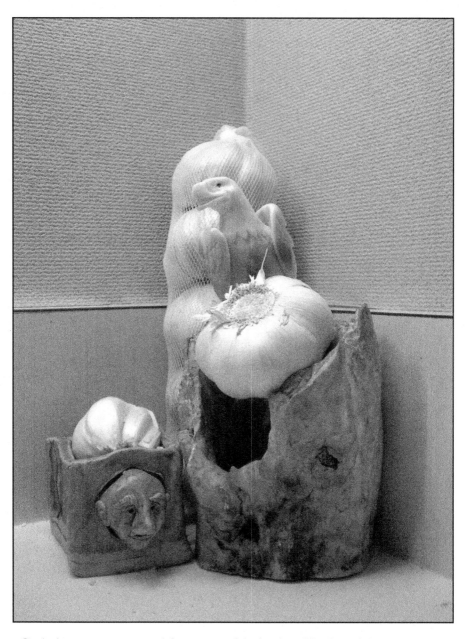

Garlic hanging out in a cool dry corner of the kitchen. Heads with large cloves are easy to peel. Increase the use of garlic and your savory dishes will grow in flavor.

14

A Well Stocked Kitchen

*S*et up your kitchen no matter the size, so you can work in relative comfort. Illuminate it. Keep it organized. Get a few basic tools. Resist filling your kitchen with gadgets, you might enjoy cooking more if you have less to clean. You can always add more depending on your cooking habits.

Consider changing shoes when you come in the house from the dusty outdoors. Don't drop off street items like a briefcase or a handbag on the kitchen counter or the dining table. Find another place for the mail. A small plant in a bright kitchen is a reminder of life. Keep an illustrated food encyclopedia[18, 19] for reference. Cultivate food literacy by flipping to a different page every time you pass by.

REFERENCES:
[18] Sheldon Margen: *Wellness Foods, A to Z*. Edited by University of California at Berkeley,
[19] Aliza Green: *Field Guide to Produce*. Their simple format and colorful plates place these two books among my favorites.

TOOLS: Invest a modest amount of money in quality cooking utensils, they could last you a lifetime. Check stores (for example restaurant outlets) that sell loose pieces rather than expensive sets. You may get lucky at flea markets or garage sales.

1. A large chopping board 12"x 18" is essential for handling large leafy greens like collards, chard, and cabbage. Keep it on the counter. Set it on a kitchen towel to keep it from moving around as you chop. If it is wood do not immerse it in water. Make sure the board is kept clean and allowed to completely air dry. Every couple of weeks rub it with edible grade mineral oil, this protects the wood from cracking and keeps flavors from penetrating below the surface.

2. A paring knife is helpful for small fruits, but to chop larger vegetables you need a sharp vegetable knife with at least an 8 inch blade. A dull knife making you push rather than slice is dangerous. The easiest way to keep blades sharp is with a sharpening stone. Hardware stores sell a block (carborundum or silicon carbide stone) for around $10. Keep it handy and get in the habit of using it once a week. Place the block on a towel and leaning the knife 20° give each side of the blade ten light passes. You will soon become an expert. (You can find helpful demonstrations on YouTube.)

3. You will value having a peeler, a grater, and a can opener. Since you will use them often, make sure they feel good in your hand.

4. You might get by without a food processor, but it is handy for lightly shredding cabbage, making date and nut dough for oatmeal cookies, mixing tofu mousse and salad dressings.

5. A simple sturdy blender great for smoothies and making soups could function as a food processor. You can find a fairly good new one for less than $150.

6. A large oven proof pan 11 x 14 x 2 inches allows you to bake sweet potatoes, pumpkins, beets, and other vegetables, all at the same time.

7. A large stainless steel bowl (15 inch in diameter) serves to soak the dirt off leafy greens like spinach, kale, and Swiss chard. Various other size bowls are good for mixing large recipes when cooking for the week or more.

8. Long handle spoon, fork, spatula, and ladle are essential for cooking in large pots. Choose an inert material like stainless steel.

9. Invest in several all purpose saucepans, pots, and skillets, at least eleven inches in diameter with corresponding lids even if you live by yourself. There is no need for non stick surfaces. Stainless steel is easier to use and clean than other ware.

10. You may end up loving a seasoned cast iron skillet. It is heavy, but heats evenly and cleans easily.

11. Invest in a dozen identical containers to avoid lid hunting. Two cups is a good all purpose size. They hold chopped ingredients and bagged lunches.

12. Don't skimp on a couple of containers with corresponding lids large enough to refrigerate your cooked beans or soups. A good size would be 8 to 12 cups.

CONDIMENTS: Buy enough for 3 to 6 months and use them while still fragrant. You will cherish spices such as cumin, fennel seeds, oregano, cinnamon, cardamom, tarragon, turmeric, pepper, chipotle, salt, and curry powders. They keep well in three ounce bottles. Group them according to sweet or savory then experiment by switching them around. Stock on olives, capers, balsamic vinegar, lemon juice, salsa, or fat free marinara sauce. A 12 ounce bottle of oil should last several months, store in a cool dark place to keep it from getting rancid. Try low fat coconut milk or coconut extract for curries and tropical flavored dishes.

NON-PERISHABLES: Buy every 1 to 3 months (in bulk if you have room to store them). Keep a variety of dry beans and lentils. Maintain a generous supply of rice, oats, quinoa, barley, and other grains. Canned beans, tomatoes, corn, and coconut milk, last many months. The same goes for cartons of calcium rich beverages like soy, almond, and rice milk which can be used in soups, smoothies, oatmeal, coffee, or tea.

NOT TOO PERISHABLE: Buy once a month. Potatoes, sweet potatoes, beets, pumpkins, squashes, garlic, and onions, keep well in a cool dry corner of your counter. Store ginger root in the refrigerator or freezer wrapped in waxed paper or plastic to keep it from dehydrating. Store extra raw nuts and seeds (like almonds, cashews, walnuts, sesame and poppy seeds) in the freezer, since their high oil content makes them prone to rancid oxidation when exposed to air and light. Consider soy products like tempeh, tofu, low salt miso paste, and keep them refrigerated.

FROZEN FOODS: Select from the great variety of frozen produce such as berries, kale, broccoli, okra, spinach, corn, and edamame. Since they thaw in a puddle, frozen foods may not be suited for all purposes. Use frozen vegetables in cooked recipes, like stews and soups; use frozen fruits in smoothies or add them to your oatmeal.

Once the kitchen is stocked, it is time to select your perishables. My patients and I have confirmed published reports that an adult can eat on $35 of fresh produce a week.

PERISHABLES: Buy every 3 to 7 days only as much as you will use, don't send money down the drain. Fresh fruits, leafy greens, tomatoes, and carrots, as well as fresh herbs and mushrooms spoil easily and must be used within a few days. Every time you shop select at least two cruciferous vegetables like kale, collards, bok choy, napa cabbage, Brussels sprouts, broccoli, cauliflower, arugula, or radishes and use at least one of them in your meals every day. Sample other delicious leafy greens like spinach, chard, and fragrant herbs such as basil, cilantro, dill, and parsley. Consider two large clear plastic bins with tight lids as extra crispers for the refrigerator. Wrap the root ends of greens, green onions, and herbs, in moist paper towel before putting them away. This will prevent too much evaporation. Buy one avocado at a time, a batch will all ripen at once. Avoid those already soft to the touch unless you like to gamble; be patient and choose a firm fruit that is uniformly green, in a day or two it will reach its peak.

SHOPPING FOR FOOD: Create a list for the recipes you plan to make that week, don't let ingredients sleep in the refrigerator without a clear purpose. Consult the section on Anatomy of Plants. Balance the big picture with texture, color, and flavors.

Explore produce stands. Take time to visit vegetable gardens. Check delivery day at your local produce market, you are guaranteed a fresher selection of greens. Explore Chinese markets and you will meet many tender and sweet varieties of cruciferous such as Napa cabbage, bok choy, and Asian mustard greens. In Indian food stores you will find a variety of rices, spices, and unusual small size dry legumes such as mung and moth beans which cook without soaking overnight. Be adventurous and try fancy dried mushrooms and fungi. A recent favorite for me is the snow fungus or Tremella fuciformis.

Freezing retains flavor and nutrition, but alters texture. Frozen vegetables and fruits (available at regular markets throughout the year) are better suited for soups, bean stews, and blends.

Resist items on sale about to spoil unless you will be using them the same day. Avoid impulse buying or buying when hungry. We bite more than we can chew. Don't buy excess, instead replenish perishable ingredients regularly.

Revise your plan when it gets stale. Stay out of ruts.

Price Look-Up codes are commonly called PLU codes. These identification numbers are affixed to produce in grocery stores and supermarkets to make check-out and inventory easier, faster, and more accurate. Currently in the 3000–4999 range this code may be a four-digit number identifying the type and variety of conventionally grown bulk produce with a voluntary fifth digit used to identify the product as organic (prefixed by a 9) or genetically modified (prefixed by an 8). For example the PLU code for regular steel cut oats is 5905; for an organic avocado it is 94225; for genetically modified foods good luck, since many growers don't want to advertise such contended qualifier on their produce.

COOKING MEALS: The kitchen is a dynamic place not a warehouse. Its vitality depends on turnover. Plan menus with the people you share meals. Include serious but playful discussions on nutrition, budget, health, and division of labor. This give and take will pay off when sitting together at the table. Meals are more likely to succeed if everyone is invested, even if you have the final say. Plan a cooking day with your home team. Anticipation makes the project grow fonder plus it will give the fruit a few days to ripen. If the family cannot possibly get together to cook, many ingredients lend themselves to advance chopping. Individuals could do prepping on their own time and still be part of the process. Save cut up food in containers (like restaurants do) until the day you will cook. As you prepare soups and stews, freeze individual portions in the same containers then use them for the lunch box and the weeks ahead.

EMOTIONS: Food is tied to traditions, security, family, and status. It expresses love and appreciation. Certain foods take on religious, political, and environmental significance. Phrases like guilty pleasures, secret stash, comfort food, or heavenly ambrosia, give away the fact that we satisfy more than our nourishment with foods. Keep this in mind as you try to change your habits.

PARTY RUTS: Revamp party trays. Present the mushroom pâté on crispy slices of raw kohlrabi or crunchy jicama. Wrap asparagus tips in thin slices of fresh ginger. End with a fragrant offering of small date and nut balls mixed with cocoa and orange rind arranged in a pyramid. (See Recipes)

HOME COOKING WITH WHOLE INGREDIENTS: Think of how many of your ingredients come out of a bag, a bottle, or a box. Try mashing potatoes or beans instead of using flour to thicken a sauce. Try frozen fruit instead of sugar in the morning oats. Try crushed apple, banana, or dates to sweeten the cookie dough. Rather than olive oil consider a mashed olive. Explore the recipes in this book and recreate your own with whole ingredients. Mustard seeds and fresh ginger impart strong flavors to otherwise bland salad dressings. The same can be said of dill or basil. Use avocado instead of oil or puréed sesame seeds (tahini) if you want an oily substitute. Process cashews with water and vinegar for a sweet and tangy creamy sauce. Add sweet dates, persimmons, or pears, to a dull dish. Make daring vegetable stir fries by adding fresh garlic, ginger, and green onion. Turn a daikon radish into spicy chips. Roast or oven bake beets, sweet potatoes, squashes, and pumpkins then add them in scoops to soups and stews. Blend a variety of seasoned cooked grains and drizzle them with lemon juice. Discover which textures appeal to you. Experiment with spices. Sample new or unusual vegetables. Taste flavored vinegars. Practice.

OUTSIDE FOOD: Once you know what to cook and how, it becomes second nature to choose nourishing food anywhere you go. Whether at a buffet, a restaurant, or a party, help your children practice this valuable skill while they are young.

TELEVISION: Most cooking shows are designed for entertainment, don't get stuck watching people cook. The web puts valuable tutorials on YouTube at our fingertips. Select an ingredient and search for recipes that use no animal products and little oil. Take advantage of the experience of others. Then practice in your own kitchen.

HAVE FOOD READY: Simple weekly food preparations allow you to pull together a whole meal in fifteen minutes. Prepare rice and beans for the week, make this your nourishing base. Store chopped onions and garlic, diced sweet red peppers, cubed potatoes, sweet potatoes, and pumpkin in medium sized containers. Rinse and spin dry a whole chopped head of napa cabbage, kale, collards, or spinach before chopping then putting it in a large sealed container for when you are ready to cook. Freeze half of your finished dishes in individual portions. Neither you nor your lunch box will ever go hungry.

Here's an easy recipe for one or two or three people:

Take out your large skillet.
Lightly cook onions and garlic in a teaspoon of water.
Add diced root vegetables and canned tomatoes and cook at medium heat for
about ten minutes until tender.
Add a large bunch of chopped fresh or frozen greens.
Sprinkle with spices, such as cumin, oregano, or chipotle and a small amount
of salt (the taste could be adjusted individually at the table).
Open a circle in the center, add a couple of tablespoons per person
of your already cooked rice and the same of beans,
and presto your nourishing dish took minutes.
Serve in wedge shaped portions to include every part of the dish.

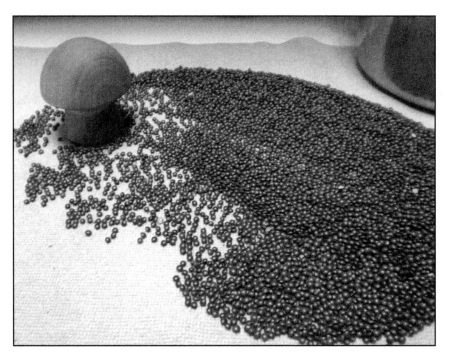

**Bags of dry legumes may contain pebbles of similar size and shape which the
processing equipment fails to weed out. Spread the dry seed, in this case beluga
lentils, over a kitchen towel and search for tooth cracking stones. Do not skip this
step. Collect this gravel in a small glass jar and display as a reminder.**

15

The Cost of Food

$\mathcal{M}$any are leaving their paychecks (a few bucks at a time) in gas station mini-marts which specialize in quick grab items for people on the run. If we insist on replacing factory foods with packaged and ready to serve produce, no doubt we will pay more. Planning a weekly trip to the produce market and time to cook could keep hard earned money from hemorrhaging out of workers' pockets. (The prices quoted were accurate at the time of publication of this book.)

CONVENIENCE COMES AT A PRICE: Eating healthier is not inherently costly, the choice is yours. Be ready to pay between $6 and $7 for a pound of prepared tabbouleh from the deli counter, or for vegetable fried rice, corn chowder, ginger and garlic greens, for a tray of sushi, or a beet salad. A one pound bag of triple washed greens sells for around $3.50. A bag of shredded cabbage and carrots costs $4. A pint of diced fruit costs $7. The price of a one ounce packet of roasted almonds is $2. In each instance you pay for twenty minutes of not washing, shredding, dicing, rolling, or roasting the ingredients yourself. Even with cut-up fruit or triple washed vegetables you may still have to put a meal together.

Buy a bunch of greens and wash out the sand by briefly dunking them in a bowl of cold water. Swish them around, pick them up, rinse the bowl of dirt, then fill it up again and repeat as many times as necessary until you run your fingers through the bottom of the bowl and feel no more grit. Now pay yourself $2 for this triple wash.

MORE ON THE MARKET OF CONVENIENCE: Buying diced fruit is expensive: an 8 ounce cup of pineapple costs almost $6, a whole pineapple a few steps down the aisle costs $3 and might fill two 16 ounce containers. Pre washed vegetables are expensive: a 16 ounce bag of triple washed salad greens can costs almost $4, a 3 pound napa cabbage sells for $3.

DO IT YOURSELF FOR A WEEK: If on the other hand you swap convenience items for whole foods, you will pay less and add the joy (or dread) of doing some cooking yourself. Buying the following whole nourishing list (prices at the time of publication of this book) adds up to about $6/day, $42/week, or $2184/year, and includes generous amounts of legumes, grains, greens, cruciferous vegetables, and fruits:

1 pound of Brussels sprouts, 28 medium size cabbages. ($2/lb)

1 pound of collards is about 12 to 16 leaves ($2/lb)

1 pound of kale equals two large bunches ($2/lb)

1 pound or a small head of napa or other cabbage 5 inches in diameter. ($2/lb = $2)

1/2 pound daikon radish 9 by 2.5 inches will slice into 27 round thins ($2/lb)

1 pound of pasta will yield about 7 portions ($3/lb)

1 pound of rice (2.25 cups dry) triples when cooked and will turn into 12 half cup servings. ($3/lb)

3 pounds of canned beans are enough for 7 portions. ($2/lb)

1 pound of steel cut oats when cooked turns into 10 servings of 1/2 cup ($1.50/lb)

5 pounds of assorted fruit will yield generous daily portions ($3/lb)

8 ounces of raw almonds serve 7 ($8/lb)

WE PAY FOR OUR DEMANDS: When we expect produce that is hard to find, out of season, or from half way around the globe, we pay for our hankering. Foods are often picked before they are ripe and travel long distances. Unnatural temperatures affect their quality even when it doesn't show on the outside. Think how many times you cut into a fine looking avocado to find dark inedible mushy flesh inside.

Informed consumers make the best of their money synchronizing food shopping with the local harvest. For example: a pint of blueberries in season costs $2 (out of season we pay over $5 and the price for frozen depends on the crop yield that year). In July one can buy an ear of corn for twenty-five cents. A couple of months out of the year sweet mouth watering mangos are almost given away. Delicacies such as asparagus are harvested over a very short couple of weeks. The price of kale stays at $2.50 a bunch, although the bunch will vary between 8 and 12 leaves. Asian markets carry daikon radish, broccoli and mustard greens, bok choi, various cabbages, and other brassica, at very reasonable prices year round. Find a good produce store and visit it often. Buy grains and legumes from bulk bins, they are usually less expensive. Keep special recipes in mind for when a coveted ingredient comes into season. Prepare and freeze stews and soups in the fall for the colder months. Turn unknown vegetables into new favorites.

LURED BY CHEAP INGREDIENTS: The price for one pound, two cups, or 100 teaspoons of sugar is fifty cents. Along with salt, this cheap ingredient is ubiquitous in processed foods. It is the main ingredient in hot lattes (popular coffee drink), water ice (a hot summer treat), ice cream, popsicles, and energy drinks. The very secret formula of a soda amounts to ten teaspoons of sugar dissolved in sixteen ounces of uniquely flavored water.

According to The Consumerist (a subsidiary of Consumer Reports blog owned by Consumer Media LLC), the average American worker today is shelling out $1040 a year on coffee—more than $20 a week, plus $1,092 on take out lunch—around $37 a week.

Compare the rounded off sticker price (at the time of the publication of this book):

Two jumbo hot dogs: $2.50; a bunch of organic kale: $2.50.
A 16 ounce bag of chips: $3; two avocados or 4 ounces of guacamole: $3.
A fruity drink: $2; a half pound of grapes: $2.

Consider whether you are buying one or many servings:

Two cans of beans or 6 portions: $3; A one pound bag of lentils or 12 servings: $3.
One glass of orange juice: $2; Three oranges to fill a glass with juice: $2.
Six packets of instant oats: $4; Three pounds of steel cut oats or 30 servings: $4.

Ask yourself if you need the convenience or are simply used to it:

A store bought cup of coffee: $2; A pound of coffee beans: $8 and 60 cups of coffee.

A case of bottled water: $5.00; Tap water: virtually free.
A granola bar: $2; Three quarter pounds of quinoa: $2.

Remember from our earlier discussions, once a kitchen is stocked with non perishable food an adult can eat fresh produce for about $35 a week.

More on the hidden cost of foods:

Two slices of pizza: $3; a couple of days of anti-acids: $3.
A weekly burger: $100 in a year; A year of doctors, drugs, and worry: $1000+.
A weekly deli meat sandwich: $100 a year; higher risk of colon cancer by age 50?
An extra 200 calories a day: gain 20 pounds in a year; 100 pounds in five.

Simple math helps us calculate how much money we spend on food and groceries, but it might be more useful to calculate the true cost that food has on our lives: How many inches have been added to our waist since age 20? How many clothes have we outgrown? How much stress have we added to our knees in the last 10 years? What is the monthly cost of our medications? Are they covered by insurance? Do we have interrupted sleep due to cough from acid reflux? Are we less productive because of aching joints, feeling bloated, or lethargic? Is sex not what it used to be? How much time are we spending at doctors appointments? Do we worry about health? Is our child's BMI (body mass index) above the expected? Is she suffering from asthma, constipation, stomach aches, headaches, fatigue, or mood swings? Everything has a price. How much are we willing to pay and for what?

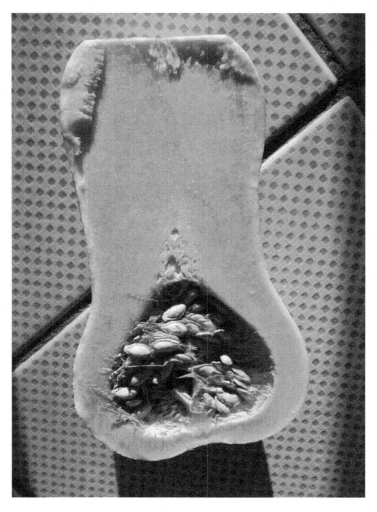

The color, taste, and nutrients of each fruit vary with the conditions in which it grew.
If you did not like the first one you tried, give another one a chance.

16

Conventional and Organic

Conventional crops grow pampered with herbicides, pesticides, and ferti-lizers. This means that they are not stimulated to produce many natural protective phytochemicals, vitamins, and antioxidants. On the other hand, organic plants grow exposed to such stresses as insects, radiation, drought, trampling, and environmental pollution. They are neither encouraged nor defended with artificial agents, so their survival largely depends on producing their own chemicals. When we make them part of our diet they also protect our DNA.

Some externally applied fertilizers and pesticides can be washed or peeled away, but not those that have become part of the flesh of the fruit or vegetable. Chemicals with a short life decompose before harvest, others last enough to land on our plate. Even when their residual effect is negligible, there are proven negative consequences to both farm worker and wildlife since at the time of application they get exposed to full concentrations of the toxic chemicals.

Competition with agribusiness is very taxing. A fair number of local growers use organic-like practices but avoid the expense of securing a certi-ficate. Get to know them. Their produce tastes better and is more nutritious. Find out more about organic farming by consulting with your area agricultural programs. [20]

REFERENCE: [20] The Rodale Institute is an organic pioneer in Kutztown, Pennsylvania. It publishes information on produce and pesticides. The Organic Consumers Association ranks the pesticides in crops and provides specific information on food and agriculture. Most state and many private universities such as Cornell, run similar programs.

It is indisputable that organic farming grows more nutritious produce and is associated with richer soil and a healthier landscape, yet the effects of eating too many calories, too much meat, cheese, and dairy, too much sugar, and too much fat, far outweigh the benefits of the obsessive pursuit of every-thing organic. We can slow down the epidemic of chronic illness and obesity by switching to an abundance of whole plants in a great variety of colors every day, trying when possible to choose organic.

Most of us not being farmers seldom think of the rich organic soil upon which we stand. When my own family started a compost pile over thirty years ago we were just curious to try it. Soon it became obvious that our fun practice was not inconsequential. We were putting out trash only every two weeks plus we were preventing barrels of kitchen and garden refuse from ending up in the landfill. We had read that compacted in airtight pockets away from oxygen most organic matter would have no chance to decompose or return nutrients to the soil. Together with how easy it was, this encouraged us to go on.

Our method was simple. We layered yard waste, fallen leaves, and kitchen scraps in a wire silo 2 feet in diameter and 3 feet tall then watched how a host of microbes, insects, and finally earthworms turned it all into black humus. We were improving a small corner of the world and it was effortless. If you are interested, check with your local township for information on composting. A short primer is included in an appendix at the end of this book.

To this day I still care for our compost pile and regularly scoop out crumbly sweet smelling black gold from the bottom of the heap.

Part III

Body Literacy

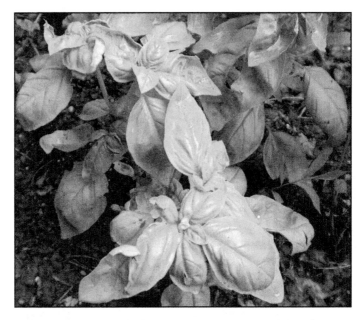

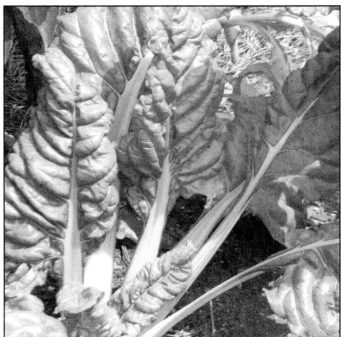

Basil and Chard are edible leafy greens easy to grow.

17

A Modern Epidemic

*A*t the time this book was published, there were 315 million people living in the USA, of which more than 30 million are obese and many more are overweight. Excess weight stresses joints especially the knees and contributes to chronic systemic inflammation. Obesity affects sleep, breathing, energy, and psychological well being. Obesity interferes with work and recreational activities. Obesity can affect the wallet, has an impact on the family, and puts a strain on furniture and car. Above all, in susceptible individuals obesity is a clear path to arthritis, diabetes, heart disease, and cancer.

Excess weight comes from consuming more calories than one could possibly use over time and represents a state of nutritional imbalance; this is true for children and it is true for adults. Fat stored underneath the skin (the fat that can be removed by liposuction) is not associated with serious medical problems other than joint stress and limited mobility. On the other hand, white adipose tissue or WAT represents fat stored within vital organs and cannot be removed by liposuction. This fat is associated with hardening of the arteries, high blood pressure, heart disease, insulin resistance, type 2 diabetes, psoriasis, cancer, asthma, osteoporosis, gastrointestinal disease, muscle weakness plus brain disorders, like Alzheimer's and Parkinson's Disease.

FOOD VENDORS FUEL EXCESS: While most people need less than 2000 calories to maintain their weight, food industries in the U.S. crank out over 3900 calories per capita. Gaining half a pound a month you could graduate from overweight to obese in five years. Markets outbid each other by offering bigger and cheaper and we subsidize them. They create false needs and we join their game. Take for example bottled water. At $1 to $2 a bottle this amounts to hundreds of dollars a year on a commodity for which we already pay to come out of the faucet and which flows free from public fountains.

The market feeds our current craze, hence ads which promote low fat or zero carbs. When the media is abuzz with gluten, even tea which never had gluten is labeled gluten free. The container must get filled, so an item low in fat is high in something else. For example: half cup of low fat Breyers Ice Cream has 2 grams of fat and 14 grams of carbohydrate. The Carb Smart Ice Cream Bar inverts this proportion with 15 g fat and 9 g carbs.

Take a look at the following examples. These items rely on simple sugars which just like fat are perfect commodities for lean times: cheap and plentiful. Highjacking our tastebuds they reel us back for more.

1. Rita's Water Ice: Serving: 12 ounces, Calories: 500, Fat: 0 g, Carbs: 126 g Protein: 0 g. Main Ingredients: Sugar and Water.
2. Gatorade: Serving: 16 ounces, Calories: 100, Fat: 0 g, Carbs: 28, Protein: 0 g, Sodium: 220 mg. Main Ingredients: Sugar and Water.
3. Fruit Loops: Serving: 1 cup, Calories: 110, Fat: 1 g, Carbs: 25 g, Protein 1 g. Main Ingredients: Sugar and Flour.
4. Juices / Refreshments / Sodas: Serving: 8 ounces, Calories: 120, Carbs: 30 g. Only ingredient: simple sugars stripped from the fiber and phytochmicals which make fruit a nutritious whole food.

MORE FOOD: The organic market section is still relatively expensive, but many stores have expanded their produce to include better quality and more variety such as kohlrabi, napa cabbage, kale, daikon radish, collards, Brussels sprouts, beets, and chard. More markets offer calcium rich non dairy milks and minimally processed soy items like tofu and tempeh. Having said that, 90% of the store is stocked with the convenience of full fledged bakeries and butcher shops plus deli meats and cheeses. Buffet style islands sell prepared food by the pound. Sweet drinks, boxed cereals, and bagged snacks have their own dedicated aisles. Refrigerators overflow with milk, cheese, and yogurt. Freezers are stacked with breaded entrées, waffles, and ice cream. It is clear where the calories pile up. As a developing country's gross national product (GNP) grows, the burden of obesity tends to shift towards groups with lower socioeconomic status (SES).

CHILDREN: The USDA encourages eating more fruits, vegetables, and whole grains. This is a tall order when cheese and chicken are fighting to stay on the plate. The existing tension between special interests and children's nutrition is evidenced in recent school lunch guidelines which see their task as limiting fat instead of increasing whole grains, legumes, vegetables, and fruits:

1. Have no more than 30 percent of calories from fat;
2. Have no more than 10 percent of calories from saturated fat;
3. Provide 30% of the Dietary Reference Intakes (DRIs) for calories, protein, vitamin A, vitamin C, iron, and calcium.

We could argue that today's children are more sedentary, spend many hours in front of a screen, are sheltered from free play, and have reduced physical activity in school, but this does not even begin to explain our predicament. The single most important change in our children's lifetime is the kind of food they are eating day in and day out. Every generation has sedentary children who prefer to read, play music, pretend with action figures, or day dream. This is the first time in our history when obesity has turned epidemic. Inactivity is not healthy, but it has not made children obese.

Furthermore, by focusing on childhood obesity as a disease of children we are making them carry a burden that belongs to adults and society. Just like we couldn't have a flu epidemic without the influenza virus, without excess calories we cannot have an obesity epidemic. From an early age children are introduced to hot dogs, nuggets, pizza, burgers, fries, candy bars, bagged snacks, juice drinks, and soda. No matter if this introduction takes place at home or at school, children have come to expect the same foods wherever they go, turning their day into a huge pile up of calories. We cannot act surprised when they complain of stomach aches, headache, and fatigue or as a result become overweight and obese.

Regularly eating from the following group of foods has made children overfed and malnourished.

Between school and home a child might eat these many calories before the day is done:

French toast sticks 2	150 calories, half of them from fat
Butter 1 tablespoon	120 calories, all from fat
Maple syrup 2 tablespoon	100 calories all from sugar
Raisin bran one cup	160 calories
Milk 1% one cup	100 calories
Orange juice 1 cup	110 calories
Pizza one slice	230 calories
Small sweet drinks 2	350 calories all from sugar
Nuggets 6 pieces	320 calories
Hot dog in a bun	270 calories
Nachos	300 calories
Cheeseburger	400 calories
French fries small	270 calories, half of them from fat
Water ice 12 oz.	500 calories, all from sugar
Candy bar	270 calories, half of them from fat

Total: 3500 calories

In contrast, the following foods from whole ingredients deliver enough energy for the day without the burden of extra calories:

Cooked Oats 0.75 cup	100 calories
Blueberries 1.25 cups	100 calories
Apple 1 medium	100 calories
Carrots/Pumpkin 1.5 cups	100 calories
Corn 1 cup	100 calories
Almonds 20	100 calories, 70% from fat
Peanut butter 1 tablespoon	100 calories, 70% from fat
Tangerines 3	100 calories
Water	0 calories
Wheat Pasta 0.5 cup cooked	100 calories
Box of Raisins 2 miniature	100 calories
Broccoli 2 cups	100 calories
Salad greens 4 cups	100 calories
Kiwis 2	100 calories
Cooked Rice 0.5 cup	100 calories
Cooked Beans 1 cup	100 calories
Salmon 1.5 ounces	100 calories
Whole Grain Bread 1 slice	100 calories
Potato 1 medium	100 calories
Grapes 1 cup	100 calories
Avocado 1/3	100 calories, 90% from fat

Total: 2000 calories

Ever younger people are ill with their obesity and are having bariatric surgery. According to *JAMA Pediatrics* November 2013, weight loss surgery (WLS) in adolescents tripled between 1990 and 2003 and shows no signs of slowing down. Regardless of the impressive short term medical results of bariatric surgery, weight loss lasts on average one to two years. Permanent weight loss and its benefits depend entirely on excellent nutrition and a healthy lifestyle.

Today's obesity epidemic is unprecedented. Hospitals are upgrading diagnostic equipment to accommodate the increasing number of oversized patients. Around 2010 Plymouth Ambulance in the city of Philadelphia was one of the first to buy an expensive bariatric ambulance to transport patients who exceed three hundred pounds. Airplanes provide routine seat belt extensions. Waiting rooms are replacing armrest chairs with sofas. Customers of institutions such as schools, workplace, hospitals, group homes, prisons, or the like, where food contracts are given to the lowest bidder, are at a huge disadvantage. Leadership together with rank and file must work on a new vision.

EATING TOO MANY CALORIES HAS CAUGHT UP WITH EVERYONE: Senior Centers offer adults in the community daily amenities such as exercise, various classes, social support, entertainment, and food. Senior Residential Homes offer all this plus health care in a permanent living facility. Meals on Wheels programs bring home-delivered or congregate meals to 2.5 million seniors; 60% have between 6 and 14 chronic health conditions and 51% take 6 to 23 medications daily.

DECEMBER 2014
Meals on Wheels

Each meal served with
Bread w/Margarine & Milk or Juice

Sun	Mon	Tue	Wed	Thu	Fri	Sat
Menu is subject to change	1 Hamburger, Tomato, Macaroni Casserole Spinach Dessert	2 Roasted Pork Ranch Potatoes Glazed Carrots Dessert	3 Creamy Chicken Corn Bread Green Beans Dessert	4 Beef Enchilada Spiced Beets Dessert	5 Rosemary-Balsamic Pork Spanish Rice Fried Cabbage Dessert	6
7	8 Parmesan Chicken Sweet Potatoes Spinach Dessert	9 Baked Fish Herb Rice Mixed vegetables Dessert	10 Meatloaf AuGratin Potatoes Cauliflower Dessert	11 Thyme-crusted Pork Roast Creamed Corn Stewed Tomatoes Dessert	12 Cabbage Roll Carrots Dessert	13
14	15 Creamy Herb Chicken Sweet Potatoes Green Beans Dessert	16 Beef Béarnaise Scallop Potatoes Beets Dessert	17 Pork with Apples Roasted Potatoes California veggies Dessert	18 Chicken Alfredo Noodles Spinach Dessert	19 Bar B Q Pork Baked Beans Carrots Dessert	20
21	22 Swedish Meatballs Rice Green Beans Dessert	23 Apricot Chicken Tomato Parmesan Gratin Cream Peas Dessert	24 Beef & Noodles Broccoli Dessert	25 *Merry Christmas* *Ham* *Green Rice Casserole glazed carrots Dessert*	26 Chicken with Rosemary Sauce Stuffing Normandy Veggies Dessert	27
28	29 Baked Fish Mac & Cheese Stewed Tomatoes Dessert	30 Hot-Roast Beef Sandwich Mashed Potatoes Carrots Dessert	31 Basil-Garlic Chicken Corn Spinach Dessert	1 *Happy New Year* Spaghetti & Meatballs Italian vegetables Dessert	2 Glazed Cider Pork Sweet Potatoes Applesauce Beets Dessert	

Meals on Wheels Menu

REFERENCE: Meals on Wheels: www.mow.org

SENIOR CENTER SAMPLE MENU from a typical Senior Center—where animal products are the identifying feature of each meal accompanied by the usual limited selection of vegetables:

Main Dishes:
Broiled Half Chicken
Meatloaf
Fried Scallops

Roast Leg of Lamb
Chicken Cattatoire
French Dip Sandwich
Chipotle Lime Tilapia

Side Dishes:

Sunday: Mashed Potato, Home Fries, Asparagus Spears, Dinner Roll,
Assorted Desserts
Monday: Tomato Soup, Scalloped Potato, Baked Potato, Succotash, Yellow Beans,
Cranberry Bread, Hot Fudge Sunday
Tuesday: Cream of Asparagus Soup, Baked Sweet Potatoes, Roasted Red Bliss, Peas
& Mushrooms, Green Beans, Onion Roll, Cream Puffs
Wednesday: Chef's Choice Soup, Rice Pilaf, Mashed Potato, Corn,
Mixed Vegetables, Pecan Roll, Coconut Cake
Thursday: Boiled Potatoes, Mashed Potato, Peas & Carrots, Lime Beans,
Dinner Roll, Assorted Cakes
Friday: New England Clam-Chowder, French-Fries, AuGratin Potato,
Bean Blend, Orange Beets, Dinner Roll, Banana Cream Pie
Saturday: Chili Beef Soup, Mashed Sweet Potatoes, Herbed Rice, Cream Corn,
Cauliflower, Dinner Roll, Jell-O

SENIOR RESIDENTIAL COMMUNITIES: Many seniors are able
to retire into independent living communities where among other valuable
services they enjoy a comfortable dining experience. However, eating restaurant style every day the weight of the average resident creeps up. It is not
uncommon to have folks gain ten to thirty pounds their first year and have
overweight added to their list of medical problems. Regardless of the excellent
medical support in such facilities, extra weight elevates blood pressure and
blood sugars, decreases stamina, and stresses joints, especially the knees. Many
facilities have contract with the same companies that serve school lunches and
except for presenting the foods in adult menu style, it is just as heavy in meat
(for example: steak, bacon, breaded chicken), cheese sauces, and processed
sweets. Seniors need a balance of nourishing plant foods with enough calories
to keep them from unintentionally losing weight. Gaining unwanted weight
represents a failure of this mission.

THE PSYCHOLOGY OF DEPRIVATION: Unless we are crossing the dessert or on a jungle expedition, we are never too far from food or drink. Constant drinking and snacking blunts thirst and hunger which are life saving body sensations. Listen to your body for signals. Step out of this vicious cycle. Trust your body again. Eat and drink on purpose based on true need.

Some people associate being thin with poverty, famine, or scary diseases, like cancer, tuberculosis, AIDS, and anorexia and worry about thin children (previously known as normal weight children).

Being under stress, without a job, short on leisure, deprived of love, recognition, money, or acceptance, all can unleash sensations similar to being hungry for food. Try to sort out these feelings.

Deprivation does not protect against excess. Take for example: sports celebrities who earn millions of dollars in a few years only to be bankrupt in a few more; or immigrants new to abundance who in the first year in the U.S. gain 20 to 50 pounds of excess weight. Having too little does not prepare anyone to deal with tempting offers such as all you can eat buffets, double cheese pizzas, or super sized drinks. Nothing inoculates one against needless consumption. We live in a culture where an avid consumer wears the twisted crown of success.

CURBING EXCESS: The key to curbing excess is in being mindful. Outlet stores offer incredibly low prices for some items, but lure you into many unnecessary processed foods. The savings in shredded cabbage might get cancelled by a box of cookies or a jar of nut butter. Make a list before you go shopping and keep to it.

Whole fruits pack nutrients, vitamins, minerals, phytochemicals, water, and fiber, all inside a unique and often edible skin of antioxidants. Factory processing changes an orange, an apple, or a handful of grapes into a marketable snack such as jam, apple sauce, or fruit leather; or else return us the fruit as juice with added calcium, some of the vitamins, and twice as many calories. A whole fruit is already great nourishment, convenient and inexpensive, nature's perfect snack.

PEOPLE WHO DON'T EAT ANIMALS: For many different reasons about one percent of the U.S. population has stopped eating foods of animal origin, but being vegetarian or vegan is not automatically synonymous with good health. People who replace meat, milk, butter, cheese, and eggs, with factory foods replete with oils, sugar, and flour, still invite high cholesterol, elevated triglycerides, diabetes, heart disease, obesity, and cancer. Mock meats (tofu turkey, wieners and burgers), non-dairies (ice cream, cheese, mayonnaise, and yogurt), pastries (cookies and cakes), and fried salty vegetarian snacks, are not health foods. Besides being high in calories they lack the water and fiber that would make us feel satisfied with a smaller portion. On the other hand, people who transition to a plant based diet quickly lose excess weight and drastically reduce their health risks. (For this reason I prefer the term plant eaters to vegetarians or vegans.)

A COMPARISON OF PROCESSED FOOD / CONVENTIONAL AND VEGAN:

1. A slice of American cheese delivers 70% of its 60 calories from fat. A slice of vegan cheese is 50 calories and still 70% fat.
2. A five inch hot dog has 140 calories, 80% from fat. Popular vegetarian wieners have 110 calories, 49% are from fat.
3. A slice of cheese pizza has 275 calories, 33% fat. A slice of thin crust no cheese tomato pie has 135 calories, 24% fat.
4. In a single hamburger there are 200 calories, 55% of which are fat. A soy burger could be 120 calories and 33% fat.
5. An 8 ounce slice of cake, whether it is regular or vegan, packs about 400 calories.
6. Pretzels, donuts, pastries, crackers, cookies, cakes, and bagels deliver too many calories often along with fat.

Here's a story to illustrate the current predicament: Our son was thirteen when we hosted an exchange student who stayed with us for a year. G. attended public high school and played for the soccer team. Tall fit and athletic this seventeen year old wanted to experience the American culture, so after practice he joined his teammates for pizza and soda. Unlike students with cars, he bicycled to and from his part time job at the photo shop, but like his schoolmates he became a regular at the local Dairy Queen ice cream shop. New to such excess and amazed that boxed cereals took a whole aisle of the supermarket he sampled each one. We all ate a plant based diet in the house and our family did not gain an ounce, but he gained twenty kilos (44 pounds) insisting he would lose them once he got back home, and he did. His saving grace was that after a brief one year experience in the U.S. he returned to a country with reasonable and disciplined eating patterns. Most people living here are already home.

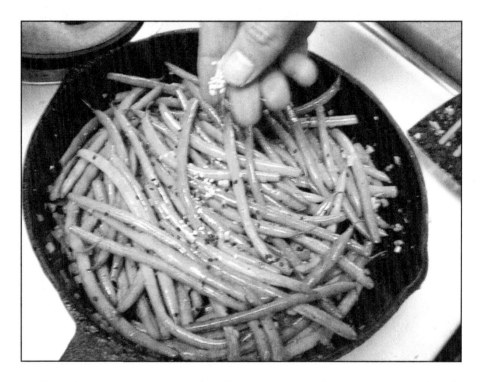

Green beans stir fried with garlic and ginger preserve their color when cooked in an open pan for just five to ten minutes.

18

The Hunger and Obesity Paradox

*H*unger is a life saver, it signals that we are getting low on glucose (our fuel) and need to find food. If we are hungry but don't eat right away, a form of emergency glucose called glycogen kicks in. If we exhaust our liver and muscle glycogen stores and remain hungry, the body begins to burn stored fat and lose weight. So, where does obesity come in?

Let us try to understand this: In 2012 about 17 million American households suffered from food insecurity, which means that 14% of families couldn't count on adequate and nutritious food consistently throughout the year. At the same time the annual per capita food production in this country is 3900 calories or 1900 calories in excess of what anyone needs. This means that many people without access to wholesome fare are never far from cheap high calorie processed food (such as sodas, pizza, hot dogs, nuggets, and donuts) and begins to explain how only 2% of the population is underweight (BMI under 18.5) while over 60% is overweight or obese (BMI over 25 and 30). Hungry people instead of burning stored fat and getting thin, can put on weight and stay malnourished.

Much of this country's overflow of high calorie food is funneled to people with limited access to nutritious alternatives. Low cost school lunches (discussed later in the book) are embarrassing. Community food pantries and senior centers are dumping grounds for commercial bakeries offering trucks full of surplus breads and pies. Many civic organizations addressing hunger in the community accept whatever. Typical items include macaroni and cheese, pork and beans, canned beef, instant potatoes, peanut butter, boxed cereals, canned tuna / salmon, canned fruit in syrup, juice, pastries, and the ubiquitous bread. Soup kitchens (check local menu) serve many patrons who depend on them day in and day out. The vulnerable among us need daily nutritious food the same as everyone else. Charities could restate their mission: to not just feed, but also to nourish and reduce diabetes, hypertension, blood lipids, cancer, and obesity; to arrest the cycle of poor health through better nutrition.

It would be easy to educate caring donors. Suggest they bring bagged grains (e.g. oats, quinoa, rice, barley); dry or canned legumes (such as lentils, beans, chickpeas); whole nuts (e.g. almonds, walnuts); and calcium rich plant milks (like soy and almond). Consider posting or mailing a letter such as this:

> Dear Donor,
> We are consciously trying to stock our pantry with more nutritious food items, therefore we will no longer accept breads, pies, muffins, or cakes.
>
> Please consider any of the following:
>
> Oats: steel cut, traditional Quaker, quick cooking, or unsweetened instant oat packets.
> Dry beans, lentils, brown rice, quinoa, barley, mushrooms, soy flakes, bagged or bulk.
> Canned beans in water, nothing added.
> Canned diced, crushed, stewed tomatoes, canned corn or pumpkin, no salt and no sugar added
> Marinara pasta sauce, no oil added
> Raw almonds, walnuts, cashews, pistachios, no oil or salt added
>
> Thank you for helping us protect the vulnerable among us.
> The Management.

Look for websites with nourishing recipes appropriate for large venues. We either pay now for oats, pumpkin, Brussels sprouts, rice, and beans or later with kidney dialysis or an admission to the coronary care unit.

Humans are omnivores which means that we will adapt to eat almost anything, it does not mean that we prefer junk food. We get used to what is available and even train our taste buds to ignore whether it's nutritious or not.

Hard pressed to eat a pound of cooked whole grain such as wheat (350 calories), we could easily finish a three ounce bag of pretzel twists (350 calories) or a large bagel (350 calories). Consider a more nutritious sampling for the same number of calories: Half a cup of cooked rice (about 100 calories). A cup of cooked beans (150 calories). Two cups of shredded cabbage (45 calories) plus a small sliced apple (55 calories). Season it with rice vinegar, salt, pepper, and mustard seeds, combine them all and you have a meal (350 calories) loaded with nutrients, fiber and water, very low in fat, sure to satisfy your hunger and keep you energized for hours.

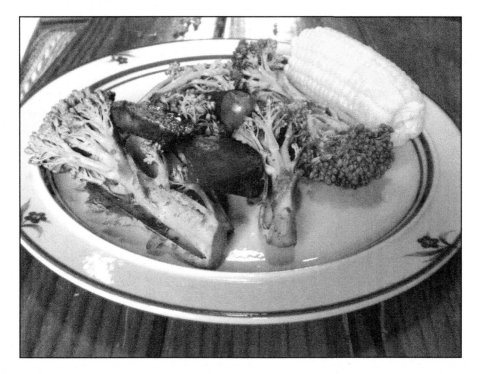

A simple summer dish—tender broccoli, baked red beet, and steamed fresh corn.

19

Exercise, Weight, Calories, and Other Measurements

Staying involved in regular exercise, not smoking, practicing some kind of meditation, and eating a nutritious diet, contribute to our wellbeing and are the best protectors of our health. We often use indirect markers such as weight, waist, BMI, intra abdominal fat, and laboratory tests, to help assess a person's health status.

PHYSICAL EXERCISE: Exercise feels good, increases endurance, helps circulation, and improves insulin sensitivity. Exercise makes us robust and builds muscles. When exercise is weight bearing it gives bones a reason to stay strong and flexible protecting us from osteoporosis. Exercise which incorporates balance and strengthens our core makes us less prone to falls and fractures. These side effects alone could encourage a lifelong commitment to the cause.

In addition, many people take up exercise with the purpose of losing weight. Why don't they succeed?

Exercise unquestionably burns calories, however it is not the most efficient way to lose weight. Without changing diet one must jog a mile a day for seven days to lose one pound. By comparison one could lose a pound in a week by consuming 500 less calories every day—the equivalent of a 16 ounce caffè latte and a bagel. Exercise is not only an inefficient way to produce significant weight loss, we often sabotage our exercise with a snack, a drink, or a post exercise reward.

Study this review: Dietary carbohydrate from plants or processed food turns to blood glucose which is our primary fuel. As exercise uses up glucose naturally its blood levels drop and we call up our glycogen reserves, which is the way glucose is stored in muscle and liver. If we continue to exercise past thirty minutes these glycogen stores get depleted and we begin to mobilize fat which is our alternate fuel. In summary, our circulating glucose together with our emergency glycogen are enough for about thirty minutes of exercise. We will use stored fat only after we have exhausted these two—first glucose then glycogen. If we refuel with food or drink around the time of exercise, we will increase circulating glucose and it will not be depleted so quickly, but if the goal was to burn fat we have defeated our purpose.

Let us continue the above story for the sake of completion. People who are starving in extremely deprived conditions are barely eating enough calories, therefore they have no stored emergency glycogen. This is true hunger. After burning what they can from a meal they still need more energy, so they go straight for the body fat; first using the fat pad behind the eyes making them sink in their sockets and so on. Eventually with little fat left to spare they will have to use a critical fat pad which protects internal organs such as the kidneys. A body in such vulnerable state is finally obligated to burn muscle just to carry out normal activities and the person loses precious mass. You could say that with no more logs to throw in the fire, we will burn down the furniture and finally the house.

WEIGHT: Weight by itself is not a indicator of health although lightweight folks tend to use less medications, suffer fewer chronic symptoms, and live healthier lives. Many people gain weight as they age, however it is not normal. Becoming overweight and obese is the result of excess calories stored as fat (true for children and true for adults). Odds are the weight you carried at age twenty suited your frame, so you could use this weight as reference even if your diet then was not the best. No matter your age now, aim to attain your ideal weight with excellent nutrition then keep it for life.

If you were an overweight child or adolescent and cannot imagine a healthy weight for your frame then the following formula could give you an idea. It yields numbers lower than expected, but it is a good place to start.

WOMEN: Assign 100 pounds for the first five feet and five pounds for each additional inch. (For example: 120 pounds for 64 inches equals 54.5 kilograms for 1.62 meters, a BMI around 21)

MEN: Assign 106 pounds for the first five feet and six pounds for each additional inch. (For example: 145 pounds for 69 inches equals 66 kilograms for 1.75 meters, a BMI around 21)

Post a picture of yourself at an age when you felt healthy, comfortable, fit, happy, handsome, and beautiful. How does it compare with the picture of you today? How many symptoms have you accrued? Are you willing to restore your health and feel like that person again? Are you willing to nourish your health and recover your body? If that is your goal, it is closer than you think.

We may be talking weight, but the objective is to be nourished with excellent food and the reward is to feel well. Childhood, pregnancy, illness, or accidents, place temporary special demands on our bodies. During such times it may be important to consult with a professional to chart a healthful nutritional plan.

BODY MASS INDEX: BMI is the ratio between weight and height, so it applies to people of all sizes, from small frames to big bones. (See Table) An adult with a BMI in the green range between 18.5 and 25 is considered normal; an adult with a BMI in the yellow range between 25 and 29 is considered overweight; and an adult with a BMI 30 or higher is considered obese. If the extra weight is carried around the waist one has a higher risk for heart disease and other chronic illnesses. However, not all high risk people have a high BMI, the acronym TOFI (thin on the outside fat on the inside) was coined to describe people who appear slender and have a normal BMI, yet have increased fat in their abdominal organs reflecting a diet that is perhaps low in calories but where those calories come disproportionately from saturated fats and processed foods.

CALCULATING BMI / EXAMPLES:

English System: uses weight in pounds (lb.) and height in inches
$$[\text{Weight} \div (\text{Height})^2] \times 703 = \text{BMI}$$
$$[150 \text{ lb.} \div (65 \text{ in})^2] \times 703 = [150 \div 4225] \times 703 = 0.0355 \times 703 = \text{BMI } 25$$

Metric System: uses weight in kilos and height in centimeters
$$\text{Weight} \div (\text{Height})^2 = \text{BMI}$$
$$80 \text{ kg} \div (1.60 \times 1.60) = \text{BMI } 31$$

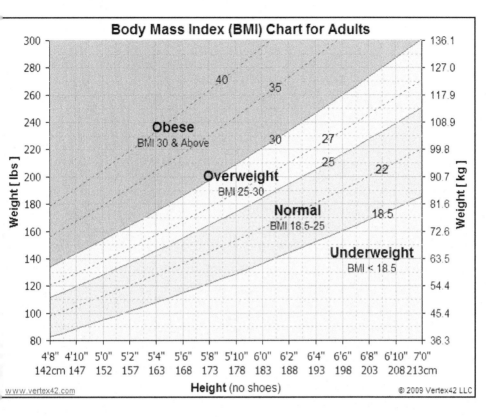

Body Mass Index

CHILDREN'S GROWTH CURVES, BMIs AND PERCENTILES: Children establish a personal growth pattern during the first year of life and usually follow this curve until around age eighteen. A child growing along his or her growth curve is eating enough calories (no more and no less) therefore is consuming enough protein. While the BMI chart for a child (just like for adults) compares weight for height, percentile charts used by schools and doctors compare BMIs of children of the same age and sex. Tragically, as overweight and obese children become the norm the percentiles also shift, so that today when we compare children of the same age and sex the overweight would appear normal and the slender underweight! Parents have a right to protest labels imposed on their children especially when schools have not instituted effective programs to support health and wellness.

WAIST: This measurement gives us another partial snapshot of our health. Measure your circumference by bringing the tape around your waist just above the hip crest and level with your navel. Make sure it is parallel to the floor and not too tight. Don't hold your breath. The adult waist should measure less than half of one's height (top limit of 35 inches or 89 centimeters for women and 40 inches or 101 centimeters for men). The larger the waist, the greater the risk that excess fat is being stored inside the liver and other vital organs. This fat cannot be removed by liposuction, but can be mobilized by eating less calories!

METABOLISM: Don't blame your weight on your metabolism. Research shows that diet resistant people unconsciously underreport their food intake by 47% and overreport their physical activity by 51%. You can imagine how this distortion albeit unintentional could interfere with the implementation of any health plan. A spotter, someone who can observe and report objectively on your food and exercise, could prove very helpful. In addition, take the Virtual Kitchen Tour and uncover calories hidden in plain sight. Most of all stop lamenting why you are not like your thin brother, sister, or friend, each of us is different. We are made to succeed, find out how you can.

FAMILY TREE: Check your family tree. Conditions that run in families (such as obesity, diabetes, hypertension, heart disease, migraine, arthritis, knee problems, acid reflux, constipation, high cholesterol, Alzheimer's, and cancer) could be fueled by diet. If you are from a family where disease genes are not easily turned on be happy, but don't assume your children will be so lucky. Help them develop good eating habits.

CALORIES: A calorie represents the amount of energy we can extract from metabolizing one gram of a nutrient. Nutrients are expressed in calories per gram:
A gram of carbohydrate generates 4 calories;
A gram of protein 4 calories;
A gram of fat 9 calories;
A gram of alcohol 7 calories;
A gram of fiber 2 calories.

The commonly accepted proportion of nutrients for our diet is 70% carbohydrates, 10% protein, and 20% fat. The Nutrition Food Label uses 2000 calories as baseline, but this is neither the average nor the goal, this number is merely an agreed convention for easy calculations. There is no typical person; an individual's daily calorie requirement is unique. In other words, adjust your intake for the desired results.

PRACTICE EXERCISE: Grab a pencil and practice how to convert calories to grams and grams to calories. This first table uses 1000 calories as baseline and you can adjust up or down depending on your needs:

1000 calories multiplied times 0.70 (70%) = 700 calories,
which divided by 4 equals 175 grams of carbohydrate;
1000 calories multiplied times 0.10 (10%) = 100 calories,
which divided by 4 equals 25 grams of protein.
1000 calories multiplied times 0.20 (20%) = 200 calories,
which divided by 9 equals 22 grams of fat.

For 2000 calories you need 100% more or double the above amounts.

For 1500 calories you need amounts halfway between 1000 and 2000 (1050 calories of carbohydrate; 150 calories of protein; 300 calories of fat).

For 900 calories you need 630 calories (157 grams) of carbohydrates; 90 calories (22 grams) of protein; and 180 calories (20 grams) of fat.

For each pound of body weight we need about 15 calories. This means that to maintain 120 pounds we need about 1800 calories. It is important to remember that extra calories carry over (like minutes on your cellphone) and it does not matter if they came from chicken, bread, water ice, latte, or beer, they catch up with us.

Eating the same, but no longer active in team sport, jogging, or the gym, the former athlete tends to gain weight. It is simple mathematics: for every 3,500 unused calories you add one pound. Tables adjusted to your level of activity help calculate your needs, however the most reliable measure is in yourself. Do not ignore the scale. No matter what any table says, if you have a surplus of unburned calories and you have gained pounds as a result, they simply won't go away until you use them.

FAT: Soaking bread in olive oil is a sure way to unconsciously pick up a few hundred calories. Since fatty foods have little water, we consume too much before feeling full. Plants (except for nuts and seeds, avocados, soybeans, coconuts, and peanuts) are low in calories and have a near perfect combination of vitamins, fiber, and nutrients.

ALCOHOLIC DRINKS:

Wine 5 ounces = 100 calories.
Beer 12 ounce glass = 120 to 200 calories.
Liquor 1.5 ounce single shot = between 115-200 calories.
Gin and tonic = 280 calories.
Frozen creamy drinks = over 800 calories.

Consider this scenario at the local pub: Alcohol is very toxic and the body wants to get rid of it fast. Your liver filters it from the blood and converts it into acetate. Easy to metabolize, acetate becomes the prefered fuel at the moment. Having enough calories from the alcohol signals the nuts and nachos that they are not needed for energy, so they get stored as fat. This is how our formerly thin and athletic college friend developed a beer belly. Is alcohol interfering with your efforts to maintain a healthy weight?

Incidentally, since your liver can metabolize only a predictable blood alcohol concentration per hour, the time it takes for your blood alcohol to return to zero depends on the amount consumed and your body weight, which for one drink may be one to three hours depending on your size. Consult tables that calculate hours to zero blood alcohol levels.

HEALTHY WEIGHT: The way we maintain a healthy weight is the same way we maintain a healthy bank account. We keep a balance between money saved and money spent; calories consumed and calories burnt. Weight Watchers, with over one million members getting on the scale each week, is by far one of the most popular and long standing diet programs in the country [21]. Its weight management is based on the correct idea that when you consume too many calories you gain weight; therefore fewer calories helps one lose weight! Subscribers use a system of points (Weight Watchers way of counting calories). However, for the most part the points disregard the nutritional quality of the food and people are not encouraged to adopt an overall wholesome diet that could serve them for life. Although some achieve and maintain their goals, most get stuck in endless cycles of losing and gaining weight as they go on and off the diet. It cannot be stressed enough that our weight should reflect a healthy nutrition and lifestyle. (See Gallbladder Disease.)

REFERENCE: [21] Nina Cherie Franklin, PhD: *Five Reasons Why Weight Watchers Fail.*

HEALTHY NUTRITION: In this chapter we have been going on and on about weight, calories and other measurements for the purpose of literacy. Once you know how to deconstruct the food on your plate, how it is that you gain and lose weight, and the various ways in which your body shows it, you can dispense with numbers and scales to be guided by your own internalized wisdom. Learning to play a song, drive a car, do math, or cook, often starts with a sheet of music, a manual, a set of rules, or steps to follow. As we practice we let go the training wheels and become free to express ourselves in our new medium.

REVIEW: Let's say there are four servings in a bag of cookies with the typical ingredients of flour, sugar, milk, eggs, and oil. Two cookies make a serving of 100 calories with 3 grams of oil; 3 multiplied times 9 equals 27, which divided by 100 calories equals 27% fat.

A three ounce serving of cooked tilapia has no carbohydrate. Its 100 total calories come from protein plus 3 grams of fat (30% of its calories) not to mention pollutants plus it lacks not just carbohydrate, but also the colorful rainbow of vitamins, phytonutrients, antioxidants, fiber, and water found in plants.

A three ounce serving of plain cooked chicken wings is 250 calories; 65% fat and the same as above.

Healthy nutrition is based on this simple guide: eating from the great variety of different color plants every day making sure to include cruciferous. Here are some recipes:

CABBAGE SALAD: Four cups of shredded cabbage plus an apple deliver 180 calories chock full of phytochemicals, vitamin C (a powerful antioxidant) plus fiber. Water content by weight is a satisfying 90%. Season with salt and pepper. Dress with a tablespoon of flavored vinegar plus one teaspoon of whole mustard seeds contributing 15 calories each. Sprinkle with 10 dry roasted almonds for another 50 calories.

SIDE DISH: Half an avocado. This fatty fruit is loaded with excellent carbohydrate, protein, fiber, potassium, and folate—120 calories. Skip the olive oil (a tablespoon is also 120 calories 100% fat and not much else) and drizzle it with lemon juice

BEANS AND GREENS: A cup of dry beans when cooked expands to a respectable three cups and contributes 7 grams of fiber. Half a cup or one portion of cooked pinto beans is 100 calories, 79 of them are carbohydrate and 20 are protein.

STEW: Generous amounts of kale (4 cups) with onions, garlic, capers, and tomato add another 100 nutritious calories. Combine them all with salt, pepper, cumin, and cilantro for a satisfying pot of nutrients. Serve it over a couple of tablespoons of cooked rice and you have a full meal.

SHORT GUIDE TO LOSING WEIGHT

In order to cause weight loss diets must limit calories, but without improving nutrition habits restrictive diets are unsustainable. In fact, most people who go on restrictive diets eventually return to their usual way of eating and gain the weight back. A better way to achieve and permanently maintain your healthy weight consists of eating an abundance of plants of different colors every day.

1. Eliminate meats, cheeses, and fried foods, so you can stop storing their fat.
2. Eliminate processed foods, so no more excess carbohydrate turns to fat.
3. Exercise over thirty minutes four times a week, to mobilize stored fat and use it for fuel.

Plan for success. We are in automatic pilot most of the day. Why not place visual, auditory, or tactile cues in our way? Set up rumple strips to signal you are going off course. I have seen the following methods help many people at the beginning. For example, brushed and flossed teeth put an end to a meal; kitchen lights turned off signal it is closed for the night; chimes hung at the kitchen entrance give pause to the unconscious visitor; a latched children's gate that must be undone to enter the kitchen might be obstacle enough. Plan your success.

Trivia: Muscle (whether form a human, a hen, or a cow, etc) is composed of protein, fat, and water. Fat is less dense than water, therefore when comparing two bodies who weigh the same on land, the fatter one will weigh less in water.

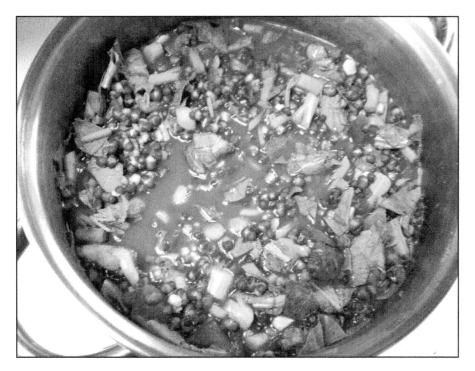

Another bean stew, this one with mung beans and young Asian mustard greens from the Brassica family.

20

Traveling the Intestinal Tract

igestion starts in the mouth. Chewing and salivary enzymes act on the food which is then swallowed slithering down the esophagus and getting dumped into the powerful stomach acid. After twenty minutes or more of churning and digestion the food bolus leaves the stomach and enters the first portion of the small intestine where pancreatic digestive enzymes neutralize the acid and are added to the mix. This is essential because although the stomach is impervious to acid it would burn the small bowel.

The pancreas has two different functions: it produces digestive chemicals that get released into the gut plus it produces insulin which is released into the blood.

Food digestion continues in a day's journey down a twenty foot small bowel tunnel spanning from duodenum to jejunum and ilium. As peristalsis slowly moves this semi liquid bolus, nutrients cross the intestinal walls and get absorbed into the bloodstream. Just at the junction of the small and the large bowel we find a vestigial no longer functional three inch long tripe known as the appendix.

The bacterial count in the dynamic nutrient rich small intestine is very low, but when the bolus arrives at the large intestine or colon it meets the largest ever population of friendly microbes (100 trillion). During the last five feet of intestine these microbes perform digestive functions otherwise humanly impossible, such as the fermentation of plant fibers that supply essential nutrients to the cells lining the colon.

After most nutrients are removed we are left with large unusable food particles plus bacteria, which make up 60% of the dry fecal mass. When enough water has been absorbed from this semi liquid bolus, waste acquires its new consistency and is ready to be eliminated. The entire journey through the intestinal tract takes one to two days.

We need 30 to 40 grams of dietary fiber a day—yet meats, cheese, eggs, and most processed foods have no fiber. Waste from these foods retain little water to help move the intestinal contents along turning stools pasty or dry and traveling the large intestine with difficulty. Drinking more liquids without enough fiber in the stools to hold on to water will simply produce more urine. On diets of animal and processed foods it is common to have infrequent bowel movements and waste which is hard or difficult to pass. People know this as constipation. Chronic constipation is the most important contributing factor to the formation of intestinal out-pouches or diverticula found in routine colonoscopy.

Many remedies are sold for constipation and can be grouped in the following categories:

1. Plant fibers keep water in the stools.
2. Stimulants or irritants quicken peristalsis and make the gut push its bolus faster. (Think of irritated bowels moving so fast that they have no time to absorb water—like in diarrhea.)
3. Water will keep stools moist only if there is enough fiber to act as a sponge.
4. Magnesium—this mineral sold as a remedy for constipation is abundant in plants which is what we should be consuming in the first place, so with this category we are grasping at straws.

The intestine is more than a churning tube where foods get digested and nutrients absorbed and certainly much more than simply a twenty foot tunnel for food to pass from one end to the other. It keeps a balance between water and electrolytes. It is a sophisticated system which regulates the trafficking of macromolecules between the environment and the host through a living barrier within the wall of the gut.

The intestine is an amazingly specialized organ. Intertwined with lymphoid tissue and our neuroendocrine network together they assure a life preserving equilibrium—tolerating our own proteins and attacking foreign ones. The term leaky gut is used when this finely tuned mechanism gets deregulated and allows proteins or half proteins and molecules which should be kept out, to be absorbed into the blood stream. In genetically susceptible individuals this can result in autoimmune, inflammatory, and neoplastic disorders.

At the level of the cell membrane there are intrinsic proteins which are constantly opening and closing much like gates exposing the intracellular genetic material to our blood plasma. These gates, first described in celiac disease and seen in other autoimmune diseases such as diabetes type 1 and rheumatoid arthritis, are ruled by diet. Our disease genes can turn on or remain turned off, depending on their exposure to outside triggers. See Epigenetics. We control most of the triggers which turn on disease genes by the diet we choose. As they say, genes load the gun and the environment pulls the trigger.

Last but not least, the gut picks up on our emotions and delivers powerful signals. Some messages like salivating are easy to understand, others can take some detective work, such as: what is the situation when your mouth feels dry?, or when you get butterflies in your stomach?, or when you have a gut feeling about something? Did you ever think your intestines were looking out for you?

Part IV

Health Caring

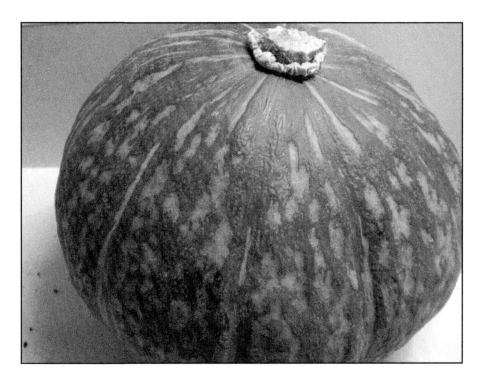

Pumpkins and squashes are fall fruits with thick hard skin which makes them durable. One could keep pumpkins and some root vegetables, such as potatoes, sweet potatoes, or beets, in a cool dry place for several months. Inside the house, their enemy is dehydration, so keep an eye on them and use before they shrivel.

21

People at Risk

*T*hree hundred and twenty million people live in the U.S. Over one hundred million of them are obese. Every year almost eight hundred thousand have their first heart attack, another half million have a second or third. Sixty-five million Americans have high blood pressure. Fifty percent of men between ages 40 and 70 experience erectile dysfunction (sign of heart disease). Twenty-million adults, almost one in ten, have diabetes. Sixty-million Americans have early stages of fatty liver. Sixty-million suffer from acid reflux, sixty-million have irritable bowel, and ninety-million live constipated. Twenty-six million suffer from asthma, forty-million have painful arthritis. Millions more have cancer, depression, Parkinson's, or some other chronic illness. Seventeen million teens have acne. Too many children are developing diabetes. Far too many children are depressed, hyperactive, lethargic, or inattentive.

We may be familiar with these statistics, but more importantly what we should know is that diet can slow down or arrest these conditions and even reverse them. Looking for a fix in fad diets, supplements, or detoxification programs people often end up throwing money away. Food has careened us into this epidemic of obesity and disease; food will pull us out of it. Once we decide to replace drugs with nourishing food a world of wellness opens up.

STATE OF OUR UNION: As this nation came out of the depression over fifty years ago, being able to gain weight was a sign of wealth, it meant that one had money to buy more. When the dust settled the bulk of cheap high calorie fast food joints had concentrated in poor neighborhoods while venues selling more fresh nutritious food settled among the privileged adding to the myth that healthy food is prohibitively expensive. Many people don't bother to plan their meals and leave chunks of their paycheck in fast food joints, mini marts, or corner stores. Exercise for its own sake, such as jogging or walking a track, is not a part of everyone's lifestyle and has added even more barriers to health and wellness. On top of that many neighborhoods lack sidewalks, night safety, well lit courts, or gyms. No one should act surprised that the poor shoulder the greatest burden of obesity.

I drive down Lehigh Avenue from the Schuylkill River to 5th Street into north Philadelphia to shop for ethnic vegetables, for art functions, and neighborhood projects. Along this thoroughfare of about thirty blocks, one end Black one end Latino, I count over a dozen corner stores selling: chicken wings and ribs, Chinese take out, bodegas of snacks and sweet drinks, pay-day lending fronts, and twice as many bars, yet not one produce stand or supermarket. Unless we understand this phenomenon of social engineering we will criticize others for overindulging or for being lazy, continue to show our ignorance, and widen the chasm between people.

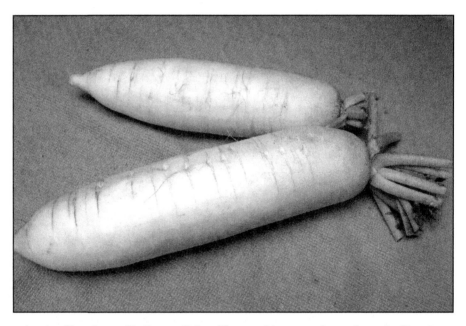

A pair of handsome Daikon radishes. Try out this unusual root from the Brassica family. Thin slices could be used instead of chips to scoop out a compatible dip.

22

Living a Solution

*I*n terms of technology the U.S. is among the seventeen most highly developed countries in the world. However, according to a 2013 report by the
National Institutes of Health, when it comes to infant mortality, heart and
lung disease, sexually transmitted infections, adolescent pregnancies, injuries,
homicides, rates of disability, and life expectancy, the U.S ranks at or near the
bottom. Why?

Advances in technology pass down from generation to generation,
but the practical answers relative to the application of technology cannot be
passed down in a formula. In other words, our decisions to where, when, why,
how much, or even whether to apply technological advances to any particular
situation must be made in the present with conscious understanding of the
immediate and long term consequences to all who will be affected. We live in
the light of brilliant scientific discoveries. We are also living the aftermath of
its many careless applications.

Regarding food, technology has allowed us to separate sugar from cane,
corn, and other whole foods. Able to amass tons of this material at very low
cost we have channeled it into our food supply just because we can and just
because it lines the pockets of dealers. It is obvious the effect this imprudent
application of technology has had on our health. Technology has also enabled
the separation of wheat germ and bran from the grain. We can grind up the less
nutritious endosperm which has longer shelf life and is more calorie dense into
a flour, and we flooded the market. This cheap product has been turned into
the every possible form of bread, cracker, muffin, pretzel, bagel, cake, pie, fritter,
and boxed cereal. Many of the surplus calories produced in this country (almost
1900 more per capita) are combinations of these inexpensive and nutritionally
boring ingredients: sugar and flour.

We can reclaim power from a food industry that has been selling us
cheap ingredients by saying I could buy pizza and soda for lunch, but I won't.
We flip the tables by saying I could go for nuggets again, but I won't. Wipe
grease off the menu. Take chicken wings and Chinese off speed dial. Instead sit

down and plan a simple menu for the week. A pot of cooked beans could get us started. In fact right now while we are thinking about it, take out paper and pen. Plan a menu and shop with purpose and less waste.

1. Let us say we want to have oats in the morning, here are some ingredients we need to have on hand: Quaker oats and steel cut oats for variety. Fruits such as strawberries and blueberries fresh or frozen and apples or grapes to sweeten the oats after they cook. Ground cinnamon (jar or bulk) makes the oats smell delicious and tastes great, too.
2. If we like rice and beans or pasta and vegetables, we need: Rice or pasta (any kind) plus large cans of beans (any kind) and vegetables for making a bean stew. Garlic, onions, carrots, sweet potato and a large bunch of your favorite green, such as kale or spinach. We like to see half the plate with some beautiful green color; fresh broccoli or Brussels sprouts taste great with some tangy seasoning. Try them with lemon juice or balsamic vinegar or with lightly toasted fennel seeds in a tablespoon of olive oil. (Although frozen vegetables retain their nutrients, in some dishes the consistency can be very disappointing.) Condiments are essential, buy them in small quantities, since they lose their attractive aroma as they age.
3. Perhaps we want to drink a cup of something hot at night, like tea or cocoa. Keep fresh ginger root to slice and steep in hot water. Plain baking cocoa powder to boil in almond milk with a teaspoon of sugar.

As we sample and sip any one of these delicious home made concoctions, we feel this is possible and plan some more.

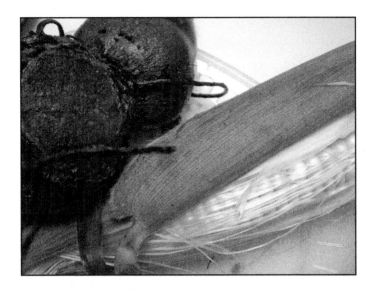

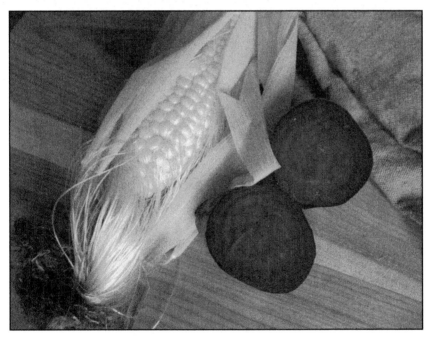

Beets and corn—smaller beets are more tender.
Bake whole at 400° for an hour then eat without bothering to peel them.
Corn picked the same day is so sweet it hardly needs cooking, but is delicious
after a short steam bath or roasted in its husk over hot coals.

23

The School Lunch Program

The U.S. government spends more than 20 billion dollars a year subsidizing wheat, soy, and corn, (and cotton—a story in itself and beyond the scope of this book). In addition, the government assists dairy and meat producers with their costs of operation and clean up. Except for cotton, most of these crops are used in animal feed or else get converted into high fructose corn syrup. The rest of these primary agricultural products are channeled into the National School Lunch Program,[22,23,24] the Supplemental Nutrition Assistance Program (SNAP), the Special Supplemental Nutrition Program for Women, Infants and Children (WIC), and the Emergency Food Assistance Program (TEFAP), explaining the presence of brand name yogurt posters in the school cafeteria, ice cream from a freezer painted like a Holstein cow, and the subsidized milk each child must put on his tray whether he wants it or not. Free water was only recently required. Most schools don't offer calcium fortified drinks such as soy, rice, or almond milk.

> REFERENCE: [22] White Paper on USDA Foods and the National School Lunch Program. On an average day, USDA Foods make up about 15 to 20 percent of the product served on the school lunch line. The remaining 80 to 85 percent is bought from commercial markets. Cash assistance for these purchases is provided from a variety of sources: state and local governments, children's payments for reduced price and paid lunches, earnings from vending machines, catering activities plus other unspecified funds available to the school's food service and the USDA.
> REFERENCE: [23] Marion Nestle: *Food Politics*.
> REFERENCE: [24] Commodity Foods and the Nutritional Quality of the National School Lunch Program. Food Research and Action Center, Washington, DC.

Sports programs tax schools with a huge ongoing financial challenge, one which cannot be met with occasional bake sales or rallies. In part to meet this demand the school lunch has been turned over to the lowest outside bidder.

The winners in this arrangement are billion dollar multinational brokers and the food distributing companies who deliver the goods. Schools boards and governing bodies are allowing the Childhood Nutrition Act to be dragged through profit driven corporate channels and are shamelessly serving cheese pizzas, frozen meat patties, canned vegetables and fruits, mealy carrots and apples, and bagged iceberg lettuce to school children.

All these brokers offer variations of the same food theme. Two common companies in the greater Philadelphia area are Aramark and Chartwells. The latter is a division of the Charlotte, NC based Compass Group and provides dining services to over 575 public school districts and private schools, comprising approximately 4,000 separate elementary, middle and high schools nationwide. The 12 billion dollar multinational Aramark provides food service to more than five-hundred K-12 school districts in the U.S. serving 340 million meals a year. In 2013 Aramark reported revenues close to 14 billion dollars. Sysco, a primary food supplier for the company which sells the same high fat high sugar processed foods to campuses all over the United States, reported revenues of 44 billion. The company offers about a dozen whole foods (for example: oats; quinoa in bulk; raw potatoes; beets and cauliflower; seedless grapes by the bunch; fresh plum and grape tomatoes; various squashes; plus minimally processed almonds and peanuts). However, since most schools no longer chop or cook on site, they order from the company's prepared menu of yogurts, ice creams, breads, pizzas, cheeses; grape based juices and jellies; with pumpkin and sweet potato appearing only canned or in pie. The company responded to a recent public demand for products from local farmers by offering the same high fat meats, eggs, and milk, from 30 instead of 1200 miles away. We are asked to accept food suppliers complaints about the added cost of training kitchen workers to handle potatoes of inconsistent sizes, a laughable excuse for not dealing with small-scale farmers.

Cheese is a staple in school. It is the country's primary source of saturated fat and is also very high in salt (NaCl). Although the recommended top limit for sodium (Na) is 2,000 milligrams a day, the industry has argued successfully that it must lower sodium content slowly over many years to maintain palatability and keep its customer base. In practical terms the school lunch is not expected to be in line with the above recommendations until 2022.

Meanwhile, each pizza pie is currently topped with one pound of cheese (7,200 mg sodium) delivering 900 mg per slice.

We should be appalled that hot dogs, burgers, meat tacos, nachos, cheese burritos, nuggets, pizza, fries, side orders of pretzel rods, chocolate pudding, and ice cream, satisfy the USDA's requirements. For extra cash at the end of the line children are allowed to buy sugar cookies and chips. Token servings of unappetizing vegetables and fruits (sliced cucumber, iceberg lettuce, baby carrots, dry broccoli florets, canned pineapple, orange wedges, corn, or mealy apples) often end up in the trash.

You may be surprised to know that schools participating in the federally-funded National School Lunch Program were only recently (starting in the 2011-12 school year) required to provide students with access to free drinking water during school meals in the location where meals are served.

The school lunch program which began in the 1940s to correct widespread student malnutrition is today a for profit business which shows little regard for the children it serves and no end to greed.

The following menus are taken from actual school websites. They represent a cross section of public and private schools from low and high income areas in the Greater Philadelphia, even though based on their food selection one could not tell the difference. When I compare them to the menus I have picked up at schools over the past few years they are mostly unchanged. I invite you to check the menus of your area schools.

ELEMENTARY SCHOOL BREAKFAST 2015

In the morning, after ten to twelve hours without food we break fast. At that time the body calls for a nutritious meal of cooked whole grain, such as oats, quinoa, millet, corn, or rice accompanied with fruit, or any combination of legumes, vegetables, and nuts. On weekends many families change the routine and serve some version of breakfast party food, such as pancakes, waffles, sausage, or a scrambler. The children who get breakfast at these schools are eating party food every day.

Monday:
Bagel with Cream Cheese

Tuesday:
   Chocolate Chip Muffin
Wednesday:
   Egg Sandwich
Thursday:
   French Toast with Syrup
Friday:
   Bagel with Turkey Sausage

Available Daily: Chocolate Chip Muffin, Fruity Cheerios, Cinnamon Toast Crunch, Fruit Loops, Frosted Flakes, Cheerios.

MIDDLE SCHOOL BREAKFAST 2014

At this school breakfast is served every day with canned or fresh fruit plus orange, apple, apple cherry juice, and milk (1%, Fat Free chocolate, strawberry, or skim).

Monday:
   Ham, Egg, and Cheese on Roll
Tuesday:
   Egg, Sausage, and Cheese on English Muffin
Wednesday:
   Egg with Bacon on a Roll
Thursday:
   Blueberry or Chocolate Chip Muffin
Friday:
   Egg with Bacon on a Roll

HIGH SCHOOL BREAKFAST 2015

Monday:
   Pancakes and Canadian Ham
Tuesday:
   French Toast Stick and Canadian Ham
Wednesday:
   Breakfast Quesadilla
Thursday:
   Cinnamon Rolls
Friday:
   Ham, Egg, and Cheese Bagel

KINDERGARTEN LUNCH MENU

At this kindergarten a child may choose a nut butter and jelly sandwich for lunch every day and no one bats an eye! She is offered a vegetable and a fruit, however mostly from cans therefore missing the opportunity to expose her to nutritious whole plant foods early in life. Even more regrettably, her young taste buds are being trained to like junk food.

Monday:
    Baked Chicken Nuggets with dinner roll
    Ham and Cheese Sandwich
    Cheese Sandwich on Whole Wheat
    Sun Butter and Jelly Sandwich
Tuesday:
    4-Cheese Mac and Cheese
    Chicken Ranch Wrap
    Cheese Sandwich on Whole Wheat
    Sun Butter and Jelly Sandwich

Wednesday:
    Hot Dog on Whole Wheat Bun
    Bagel and Yogurt
    Cheese Sandwich on Whole Wheat
    Carrot Sticks and Ranch Dip
Thursday:
    Chicken Tender Plate
    Pretzel Twists
    Turkey and American on Whole Wheat
    Sun Butter and Jelly Sandwich
    Baked Tater Tots
    Garbanzo beans
Friday:
    Cheese Pizza
    Yogurt, Veggie, and Cheese Sticks
    Cheese Sandwich
    Sun Butter and Jelly Sandwich
    Broccoli florets

ELEMENTARY SCHOOL LUNCH 2014

To accommodate all the children, many schools serve lunch in twenty minute shifts beginning at 10:15 in the morning. These heavy meals are wolfed down in a noisy unsettling environment and often result in a dip in attention and alertness for the afternoon classes.

Monday:
    Popcorn Chicken
    Mighty Macho Nachos Pack
    Chef Salad Plate
    Corn
    Broccoli tips with Ranch Dip
    Fresh Fruit – every day
    Canned Fruit – every day
Tuesday:
    Sizzling Philly Cheese Steak Sandwich
    Pizza Party Pack
    Garden Salad
    Dinner Roll
    Carrots
    Baked Tater Tots
Wednesday:
    Cheesy Stuffed Breadsticks with Marinara Sauce
    Bagel and Yogurt
    Garden Salad with Turkey and Roll
    Carrots
    Baked Tater Tots
Thursday:
    Nachos Grande with Cheese
    Turkey and American on Whole Wheat
    Chef Salad Plate
    Romaine and Cherry Tomato Salad
Friday:
    Cheese Pizza (every Friday)
    Chicken Ranch Wrap
    Garden Salad with roll
    Broccoli

MIDDLE SCHOOL LUNCH 2015

Every meal comes with milk and available daily are pizza, grill sandwiches, and deli bar. Children may also have fruit, juice, veggies, and fresh salads. However, the main menu consists of meat and cheese combinations—this even though the USDA commodities program offers to the schools a wide selection of whole foods just for the asking. Health Class teaches students food literacy and the cafeteria offers the best opportunity to reinforce this learning by feeding the children more delicious nourishing plant food. Who will go first?

Monday:
>Buffalo Chicken
>Mac and Cheese

Tuesday:
>Teriyaki Chicken with Rice

Wednesday:
>Beef Lasagna Roll-Ups with Melted Mozzarella Cheese

Thursday:
>BBQ Brisket

Friday:
>Classic 3 Cheese Pizza

HIGH SCHOOL LUNCH 2015

By the time many children are in high school their tastes are exclusively trained on fast food.

Monday:
>Breaded Steak with Roll
>Hot Dog
>Mashed Potatoes with Gravy
>Broccoli with cheese
>Cinnamon Sweet Potatoes
>Fruit Variety (every day)

Tuesday:
>Pasta Bar
>BBQ Rib Sandwich

Black Beans
Mexican Corn
Baked Fries
Wednesday:
Sloppy Joe Sandwich
Corn Dog
Baby Carrots with Ranch
Celery Sticks with Ranch
Thursday:
Oriental Bar with Kung Fu Rice
Green Beans
Steamed Carrots
Baked Fries
Friday:
Lasagna with Bread Stick
Breaded Steak Sandwich
Golden Corn
Romaine Side Salad

While it is true that some schools offer more nutritious options they are the exception, so do not rest on their laurels. I invite you to check out the menus of schools in your area. Those here displayed are the rule and have the following in common:

1. The menu of every day is defined by the meat—even when MyPlate. Gov has removed it as a food group.
2. Items shown as nutritious in wall hung pictures are not featured on the menu. (Brown rice, cauliflower, asparagus, spinach, mushrooms, peppers, cabbage, kale, dates, sweet potatoes, oats, and blueberries.)
3. Every child must take the subsidized milk with no alternative calcium rich beverages such as soy or almond milk.
4. Carrots, peas, romaine, and broccoli could be taken for the epitome of vegetables when in fact they simply come conveniently packaged.
5. Chilled fruit is served out of syrupy cans.
6. Almost every school across the nation features cheese pizza on Fridays.

Over the past few years I have visited, with my colleague Barry Jacobs and first year family medicine residents, over thirty elementary, middle, and high schools in Southeastern Pennsylvania served by different food companies. I left each one deeply saddened. Whether public or private, from affluent neighborhoods or poor, the typical menu is the same. Vending machines might be turned off during lunch, but the elephant is still in the room. Picky eaters can choose a hot dog every day for lunch or a peanut butter and jelly sandwich and no one cares. Children bringing a home packed lunch are not faring any better munching on granola bars, fruit leather, cheese sandwiches, peanut butter cups, chips, pretzels, sliced cheese, deli meats, fried chicken, salty crackers, and sweet drinks, with the occasional baby carrot, apple, or banana. Rarely did I see greens, grains, or beans. (Visit MyPlate.Gov for the most recent dietary guidelines.) On the way to or from school many children stop at corner stores for caffeine drinks and sweets.

Citing that only one in ten schools in the U.S. have the necessary equipment to cook, the USDA has offered grant money to improve the schools' kitchens.[1] Sadly, most schools contract outside providers and use their ovens and stoves merely to reheat the food. One could also assert that children and parents are used to the same convenience food in and out of school, so changing the cafeteria without first introducing nourishing foods in a supportive learning environment is likely to fail. A sensory based plant food curriculum with kitchen laboratory sessions advances food literacy and paves the way for children to accept new foods from a personal experience.[2]

REFERENCES:
[1] Press release 2014/006514. The U.S. Department of Agriculture (USDA) is awarding $25 million in grants to help schools buy needed kitchen equipment.

[1] *The Pew Trusts Research and Analysis/Collections.* 2013/12/18/serving healthy-school-meals-kitchen-equipment-collection. Only 1 in 10 school districts nationwide (12 percent) has all the kitchen equipment needed to serve healthy foods, according to a new report issued by the Kids' Safe and Healthful Foods Project.

[2] Food Studies Institute and *Food is Elementary* presents a sensory based curriculum by Antonia Demas, PhD, in over three thousand schools across the nation.

School nurses report too many children with joint pains, asthma, constipation, stomach aches, headaches, fatigue, and various attention and mood disorders, all of which can be signs of poor nutrition. Making matters worse, even though by middle school more than forty percent of the children are overweight or obese, many schools have cut back on their physical activity.

As learning institutions schools must teach the connection between nutrition and health, but reversing this trend won't be effortless or free. First priority is food literacy, among children, parents, and school officials—schools are in the best position to deliver on this, since most serve lunch and breakfast every day.

You may be tempted to think that all we need is a change of menu or to give the school cafeteria a make over; think again. In 2010, U.K. celebrity chef Jamie Oliver was appalled by the news of growing obesity among children and their poor eating habits, so he visited the U.S. determined to lead a revolution, yet no one followed. Why did he fail? Many felt that he embarrassed school officials, that he was impatient and condescending. Without a long term sustainable grass roots plan, his method felt tactless and perhaps imposing. He flunked at bringing an informed group of parents, children, and teachers along. Saddest of all, this failed public stint may discourage future efforts for years to come. Next time someone mentions revamping the school cafeteria the negative experience of 2010 will be offered as excuse to stall. How can a school get ready to adopt healthful changes? Visit the Food Studies Institute website cited above for some ideas.

PUSH AND PULL: Schools can order from a variety of government commodities (oats, rice, various legumes plus frozen fruits and vegetables). Under the existing system these commodities are handed to outside companies who return them as tray-ready food. A couple of times a year the local food trust brings demonstrations to school, but what good is this when the children are sent back to eat pizza, nuggets, chips, and burgers at the cafeteria like every other time? In a half hearted gesture before summer break, schools are encouraged to order fresh produce from area farms—this is too little too late. Why not plan an inside garden during the school year? In another pathetic display of lackluster leadership some consultants have suggested packaging apple slices and carrot sticks to look like junk food (their term not mine). We don't need to disguise whole food to make it "appealing" what we must do is teach food literacy and develop children into savvy consumers who would not be duped by mass marketing. Missing the point again, schools tend to respond to criticism by cluttering the menu with yet more choices of party foods. Where is the year long program that would teach food literacy? School officials are either afraid to take the lead or truly ignorant and misinformed. Whatever the case, children deserve better.

LUNCHTIME: It is unfortunate that in most schools teachers do not eat with students. True that the environment of most cafeterias is chaotic and loud not conducive to a peaceful meal or healthful digestion, which by the way affects children the same as adults. Peace or quiet is not attained by yelling rules and admonitions—the mood is rather set at each table as individuals consciously bite, chew, and recharge their energies with food and community. Children respond in kind when adults converse with them and care for them in respectful ways.

> REFERENCE: Teachers' contract and lunch time: What can I be assigned to do during my lunch period and my prep period? May 12, 2011 *New York Teacher* issue. All teachers have the right to a duty-free lunch period every day. You should get no assigned work during this time, including meeting with a coach. Such an assignment cannot be mandatory.

"Teachers probably wouldn't mind eating with their students as long as they were guaranteed a 30 minute duty-free slot in their day to be used as needed. Apparently that runs into all types of logistics problems. There is no "free" time other than lunch. Elementary school teachers in particular have almost no other time." —Retired elementary school teacher.

Teachers who sit down to eat with students seize a mentoring opportunity. They can cultivate table manners, have informal conversations about food and health, even discuss what a nutritious bagged lunch could look like. A civilized chat at the table does not require special preparation or a certificate— simply a genuine desire to respectfully connect with each other.

Having said that, teachers might not feel comfortable advancing food literacy. I have gone on Virtual Kitchen Tours of teachers, doctors, nurses, dietitians, lawyers, and other professionals and most suffer from the same nutritional misconceptions and imbalances as the general public and my patients.

I suggest that any questions about food and health that arise be postponed and picked up the next day after students and teachers have done some research at their own pace on their own; then together share what they found. This style of learning, rather than spoon feeding and memorization, cultivates a scholarly approach to life's questions instead of opinions that can be thoughtlessly spewed.

FOOD LITERACY FOR CHILDREN: Today's foraging grounds tend to be fast food joints, delis, all you can eat buffets, malls, and of course supermarkets where aisle upon aisle is stacked with packaged food. Too many people can spend a lifetime without knowing where their food comes from. Children growing up on fast food will hand down this ignorance to the next generation. Humans and edible plants separated by an abyss.

Imagine a curriculum where the nutrition class is taught with fragrant juicy real food instead of cardboard cut outs. When we place food (such as arugula, rutabagas, radishes, collards, bok choy, sweet potatoes, squash, rice, beans, quinoa, oats, berries, pomegranate, and avocados) in children's hands to touch, see, and smell, they are tempted to taste it without coercion. The way to teach food literacy is gently through the senses and over a long haul.

A wise selection from the free commodities foods available to the schools would satisfy calories, protein, calcium, vitamins, fiber, antioxidants, and minerals. Imagine schools with kitchen laboratories where children learn to read recipes, follow culinary steps, measure, chop, mix, and actually cook. Climate permitting, schools could tend a vegetable garden. Who knows, schools might invest in greenhouses! Children who learn how food nourishes the body grow up discerning consumers.

Peddlers of fast food and sweet drinks have taught our children to like their products. Teenagers are lining the pockets of greed with their eating habits. Young people must know how the body uses food to grow, repair, and renew itself. Families need food literacy and body literacy. Children should understand how antioxidants protect cells from unhealthy mutations and how fiber and water help rid us of toxins. Many a chapter in this book will serve this demand. Children who develop curiosity and respect for the body will protect it. Children and adults must take off their blinders, adults first.

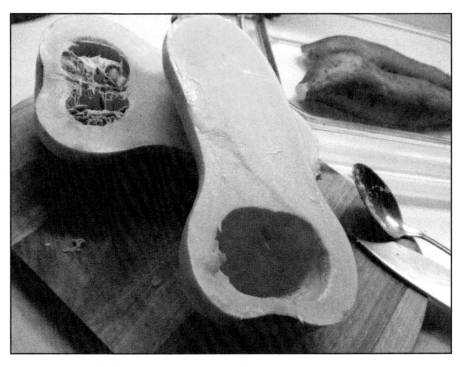

Butternut squash, sweet potatoes, and pumpkins—the carotenes almost jump out of the page. Our bodies use carotenes to make Vitamin A.

24

The Incubation of Chronic Illnesses

*W*e tend to medicate early signs of health imbalance, such as weight gain, high blood pressure, high cholesterol, or erectile dysfunction. Commonly, people live with a blind eye to the effects that diet and lifestyle are having on their health until they have a heart attack, develop diabetes, or even cancer. The expression out of the blue is shall we say an urban myth.

We put too much stock on medical tests which rather than health-preserved measure health-lost. Good health is a state of thriving wellbeing for which we have no test. Furthermore, medical tests won't detect disease until it has incubated silently for ten to twenty years. Good health is not defined by the absence of illness anymore than peace could be defined as the absence of war.

Developed countries living in abundance are disproportionately plagued by chronic illnesses, yet we share 99.9% of our genes with every other human on the planet. This means that the uneven distribution around the world of these conditions cannot be explained by genes alone.

Accumulated data show that as developing countries modernize and urbanize, people start consuming more fats, more animal based products, more sugar, more processed foods, and less fiber.

"A combination of economic and social factors is contributing to these dietary changes. One factor is relative food prices: The 20-year trend in global prices of edible oils, animal-based products, and sweeteners has been downward, contributing along with increased incomes to greater consumption of those foods in developing countries." [25]

Through this transmutation, people accrue the three main risk factors for chronic illness: over-nutrition, lack of physical activity, and tobacco use. Examples of chronic illnesses include: obesity, diabetes, heart disease, acne, arthritis, migraine, sexual dysfunction, gastroesophageal reflux, inflammatory bowel, and diverticular disease; kidney and gall bladder stones, autoimmune disorders like rheumatoid arthritis and multiple sclerosis, acquired immune deficiencies, and some cancers. Most notably, these developments following westernization are reversible.

"The alarming aspect in regard to the public health and economic agendas of these countries is the speed with which unhealthy habits have taken hold in developing countries, with little indication of slowing."[25]

REFERENCE: [25] Rachel Nugent: _Ann N Y Acad Sci_ 1136(1):70-79 (2008), PMID 18579877 Chronic Diseases in Developing Countries Health and Economic Burdens, Center for Global Development, Washington, DC, USA.

Optimal health defies being measured by the same ways we measure disease.

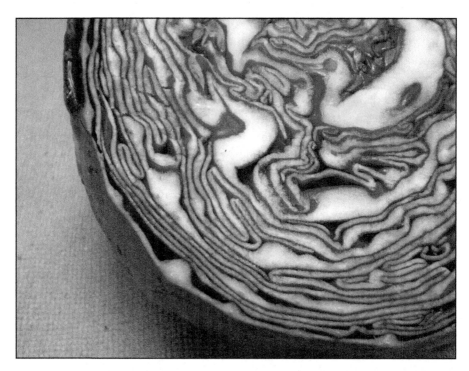

Cabbages of any color are tightly packed leafy heads from the Brassica family and much more resistant to dehydration than lettuce, spinach, or chard.

25

Inflammation and Health

*F*ree radicals are unstable atoms or groups of atoms which form when oxygen interacts with certain molecules. Highly unstable, due to its unpaired number of electrons, a free radical stabilizes by reacting with any other molecule that can lend it an electron. When free radicals react with our DNA (genetic material) or the cell membrane, they can cause vital cells to function poorly or die, so it is no coincidence that we often think of free radicals in negative terms. However, these molecules are a normal byproduct of the body's metabolism and in measured amounts play an important housekeeping role. They induce the controlled death (apoptosis) of cells that are sick, old, or have already served their purpose and precisely due to their destructive nature they help us fight infections by zapping bacteria. Think of these highly unstable molecules as guardian angels that patrol our internal environment and try to keep it clean, but which in turn must also be kept in check.

INFLAMMATION: In response to an acute injury the immune system barricades the damaged site by flooding it with first-responder cells such as macrophages and with chemicals including helpful free radicals. This response results in visible redness, swelling, warmth from the rush of blood, and often pus and pain. Acute inflammation disposes of the harmful situation by containing it. For example, in a boil the enemy (whether bacteria or a foreign body) is attacked and walled off then eventually expelled. In due time this cleansing fire cools off, tissues regenerate, and the site is healed. If the injury is serious enough, this rapid response could mean the difference between life and death.

Chronic inflammation is another story. When free radicals are spewed in sustained amounts without a target (which is the common situation on a diet of processed foods and animal products) they attack innocent tissue causing cell damage and DNA mutations. Imagine our immune system in this situation as a team of fire fighters trying to wrestle an invisible smoldering fast spreading fire by aimlessly wielding axes and hoses. The similar response by macrophages, inflammatory prostaglandins, cytokines, and interleukins which is so beneficial in acute inflammation, in this case does more harm than good. Spilling into the blood without a clear purpose, they reduce to cinders everything in their path causing chronic pain, deforming arthritis, heart disease, diabetes, cancer, and other chronic inflammatory conditions such as acne and Crohn's disease.

INFLAMMATION'S DOMINO EFFECT: 1, 2, 3

1. CHOLESTEROL fat cannot dissolve in our watery plasma, so a low density lipoprotein (LDL) must carry it and drop it inside the cells. Once a cell has accepted enough cholesterol its surface receptors shut down, leaving the exposed excess LDL-cholesterol pair to wander about in the blood. This wandering pair is easy target for free radicals, which will quickly oxidize it creating 'a situation'. The macrophage cells living within the vessel wall are important first responders to such oxidized spills eating foreign material, dead cells, and debris. In this case they fill up with the damaged fat droplets ballooning the arterial lining (endothelium) into the center of the blood vessel (lumen), changing into what we call foam cells. As foam cells get larger they stretch the vessel wall so thin that it can no longer produce nitric oxide. The arteries lose their elasticity and become stiff.

2. HIGH BLOOD PRESSURE: Having lost their ability to dilate normally the now stiff blood vessels cause elevated blood pressure. Unable to dilate normally during exercise, blood vessels have trouble delivering necessary oxygen to the tissues, which can cause intermittent leg pain (claudication) or chest pain (angina). Arteries that cannot dilate normally during sexual excitation can present as erectile dysfunction. All these symptoms are telltale signs of heart disease.

3. HEART ATTACK: Let's pick up again on the blood vessel whose lining is stretched very thin by the ballooning foam cell. With each heartbeat the inside of the arteries is exposed to swift moving blood which drags the lining with it creating a shearing effect. If a vulnerable spot in the thinned arterial wall tears open, the foam cell spills its contents into the blood and an ensuing fast forming clot interrupts the circulation. The heart muscle beyond the clot is left without oxygen and dies, in the dramatic event we call a heart attack.

Free radicals are carefully monitored by the body. When they reach excess levels a free-radical-stress-response sends for glutathione which is a powerful intracellular antioxidant and together with dietary antioxidants such as carotenes, Vitamins C and E, and other phytochemicals, all rush to neutralize the excess free radicals and repair some of their damage. If we want to move toward a healthier internal balance we need to do more than simply eat fruits and vegetables for their antioxidants, we must level the playing field. We give plant antioxidants a fighting chance by eliminating dairy, greatly reducing or eliminating meats and sweets, limiting alcohol, managing stress, quitting smoking, exercising regularly, and getting close to our ideal weight.

NUTRITION AND HEALTH: Free radicals are the product of normal digestion. They also result from the metabolism of prescription drugs and supplements, of tobacco, and environmental pollutants. Free radicals result from the metabolism of food stabilizers, preservatives, colorings, and flavorings—all of which are waste from the start.

The blood gets filtered through the kidneys and the liver many times a day. These organs in turn pour our waste into urine and bile. Produced in the liver and stored in the gall bladder the bile squirts into the small bowel where it mixes with intestinal waste and is eliminated in the stools.

Plants supply us with antioxidants that neutralize excess free radicals. The brassica or cruciferous plants besides being highly nourishing, stimulate the detoxifying function of the liver. A sampling from that group includes: Brussels' sprouts, Broccoli, Cauliflower, Arugula, Watercress, Radishes and Turnips, Daikon radish, Horseradish, Rutabaga, Napa Cabbage, Bok Choy, cabbages, Kale, Collards, Mustard Greens, Turnip Greens.

THE ROAD TO DAMASCUS (a sudden turning point in a person's life): Most people truly want to feel better, but making lifestyle changes is difficult. When we are frustrated we become more vulnerable which makes us susceptible to advertising promises. We can be tempted to try anything (anything but change, that is). However, we should keep in mind that weight loss plans and detoxification programs share statistics which are not very bright. After a few years only a quarter of participants keep off even 10% of the weight they lost. Eventually most folks resume old habits to regain their weight and symptoms.

Consider this: Eating plants rather than animal and processed food generates less waste, less symptoms, and less weight. It seems more prudent to invest the same money and effort cultivating a healthy lifestyle and if you smoke, quit.

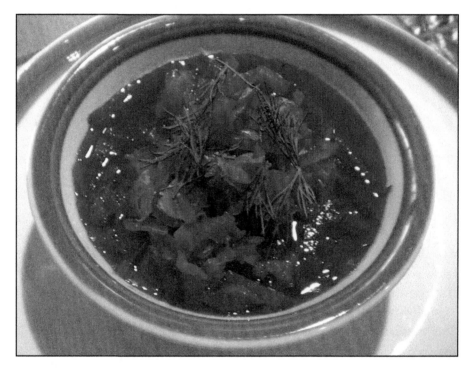

White cabbage is hardly recognized in this red beet borscht garnished with dill.

26

Sick Care Is Not Health Care

*W*e neglect taking care of our health by limiting health care to laboratory tests and medical check ups. Sick care, such as when we need treatment for an infection, emergency surgery, or for a serious chronic condition, is essential, lifesaving, and priceless—but it is not health care.

Health care is a personal practice. Eat well, exercise, work, play, relax, love, and don't smoke. Tune regularly to your body. Occasionally we pick up subtle signs or symptoms not yet dramatic, but signaling an organism under stress. We tend to neglect them because we know that a headache is hardly ever a brain tumor, that fatigue has many origins, that back ache is only rarely a herniated disc, that abdominal pain is appendicitis only once, that shortness of breath has causes other than asthma, and that every chest pain is not a heart attack. However, these vague and common symptoms are red flags and signal that something is out of balance and deserves our attention.

When you pick up on any such communication from the body, pause. Check for anything that might be within your control that could be contributing to the distress. It might be your food, lack of sleep, no exercise, or something else. Attend to it. Consider the pressures you are under. Take note of how you have put yourself in this predicament several times before.

The more health care we practice the less sick care we might need. Daily nourishing food, regular exercise, being involved in something larger than oneself, all this is health caring. Many people include walking, dancing, sculpting, painting, cooking, swimming, kayaking, cycling, composing, music, playing an instrument, singing, yoga, meditation, or psychoanalysis, in the practice of their health care. What are some ways in which you care for your wellbeing?

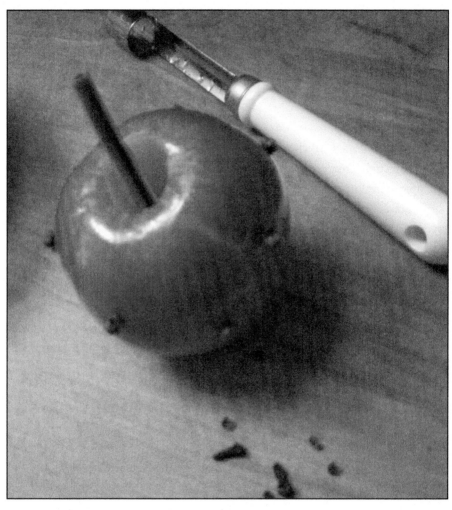

This apple studded with spice cloves had its core replaced by a cinnamon stick. It will stew with an inch of water in a covered pot for about thirty minutes when a sweet smell will permeate the house announcing it is ready.

27

Epigenetics

O f the 20,000,000 plus genes in the human DNA, only one percent of them is different among individuals. This very small fraction of genes determines unique and immutable personal characteristics such as sex, skin pigment, blood type, and hemoglobin. The rest of the DNA is a huge set of blueprints for making proteins and fats that will participate in myriad chemical reactions. These blueprints also contain instructions for diseases. However, disease genes can stay off or be turned on depending on our diet. This explains how many diseases tend to cluster in families.

Disorders determined by particular genes, for example muscular dystrophy, sickle cell, Tay Sacks, or phenylketonuria, are quite rare and affect only one out of several thousand or several million people.

On the other hand, we could say that many conditions, such as gastritis, acid reflux, hypertension, diabetes, migraine, heart disease, gout, kidney stones, gallstones, high cholesterol, colon cancer, arthritis, and obesity, run in families by way of the kitchen. Adopting a healthier diet of more whole plants and less refined flours, sugar, oils, meat, and dairy, keeps disease turned off, protects genes from cancerous mutations, and will help reverse many chronic illnesses.

The following example illustrates this phenomenon of epigenetics. In *The China Study*, Cornell Professor T. Colin Campbell, PhD, describes a certain area in China where almost all the children had been exposed to a peanut crop contaminated with an aflatoxin producing fungus. In a striking turn of events, the children from affluent families and who ate the most animal protein developed liver cancer, but the children from modest means eating a plant based diet did not. In other words it was not the toxin by itself which instigated the cancer cells, but the associated diet. His group went on to test this hypothesis and although it was difficult for him to implicate meat in such a terrible outcome, the evidence was irrefutable.

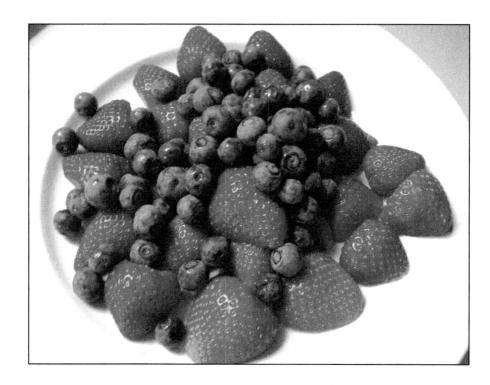

We feast on berries in season.

28

Getting Off Medications

*W*hen we ignore the host and the role it plays in the development of illness we assume that each disease is a formidable alien attack. For infections and physical injuries this model works fine, but when we try to apply this model to chronic illnesses we in fact miss the boat. The common culprit in many illnesses is inflammation from within and by allowing it to go on without attempting to halt or to reverse it we create the perfect storm.

Our medical health care system has poured enormous resources into a very specialized model of surveillance. It aims to detect manifest disease to then intervene with drugs and procedures, using the excuse that it is too late and difficult to alter diet or lifestyle. This model thrives because it assumes humans could not be disciplined and care for their health— for the most part this is a self fulfilling prophecy. Our lucrative health care model, based on micromanaging, is so intricate and complicated that once you fall in it traps you like a spider web.

Many commonly used classes of drugs are valued for their anti inflammatory properties. One of the most potent examples is steroids. In the form of inhalers and sprays they form the mainstay treatment of chronic asthma and nasal allergies. These potent anti inflammatory drugs reduce swelling, narrowing of the air passages, itching, and mucus, and do so by disrupting the inflammatory immune response.

Other common anti inflammatory and immune suppressor drugs include those used to treat Rheumatoid arthritis. Although we don't fully understand their mechanism, drugs like methotrexate and adalimumab (Humira), temporarily weaken the immune system forcing patients to choose between having less inflammation or retaining their current resistance to infections.

Like many other commonly prescribed drugs statins, whose original use was in lowering various lipids or fats in the blood, protect against disease by also suppressing inflammation.

There is no doubt that drugs reduce inflammation and damaging oxidation, however drugs are a two edge sword to be handled with utmost care. The number of deaths due to the correct use of prescription drugs in the correct dose is staggering.

> REFERENCE: *MMWR Morbidity and Mortality Weekly Report.* During 2010 (the year in which the latest national NVSS mortality data are available), a total of 40,393 drug-induced deaths occurred in the United States. The majority or 74.3% of these drug-induced deaths were unintentional.

Our mission if we choose to accept it is to reduce the need for many anti inflammatory medications by generating less inflammation. We do this by approaching disease from within, the same way it developed.

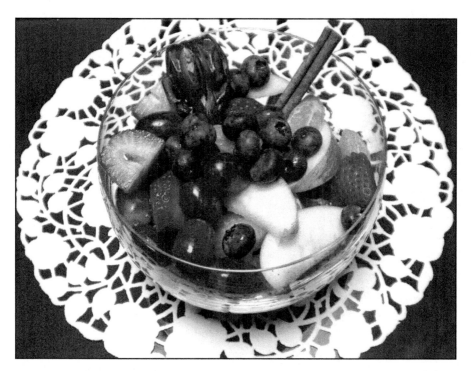

When the supply starts to dwindle, combine berries with other fruits. Here they are served with apples, grapes, oranges, and a pitted moist Medjool date.

29

Supporting a Healthy Balance

A healthy immune system is tireless. We are said to live in homeostasis, yet far from static we are dynamic, self monitoring, and constantly self-organizing. Whenever balance is threatened, internal mechanisms try to keep us from going over the edge.

Among its many tasks the immune system puts a crimp on damage done by free radicals, it looks after tumor suppressor gene p53, protects our DNA from cancerous mutations, instructs potential cancer cells to die, turns inflammation on and off, and helps tissues heal, all in a day's work. We live among myriad chemoactive substances and competing reactions. Our dynamic organism is in constant production, destruction, and repair. When we speak of the immune system, inflammation, free radicals, detoxification, or cancerous mutations, we are talking about a huge web of interconnections.

The success of micromanaging with pharmaceuticals often depends on the very precise interruption of some metabolic reaction while taking great care to protect its counterpart. For example, people on non-steroidal anti inflammatory drugs for pain and inflammation can develop stomach ulcers and bleeding. This led to the discovery of celecoxib (Celebrex), a selective drug that blocks the inflammatory effects of cyclooxygenase 2 (COX 2) while it preserves cyclooxygenase 1 (COX-1) function thereby protecting the stomach lining. The more of these biochemical reactions we discover, the more points for drug intervention we amass. There is no question that drugs can help tilt the balance in a good way, but there is a catch. Drugs have good effects and side effects. Precisely because these reactions exist interconnected every time we alter a pathway we tug at some other strand of the web. Also due to this interconnectedness, drugs do not act exactly the same way every time or in every person, at times surprising us with the opposite effect than the one we seek.

Drugs are invaluable adjuvants when health has reached a precarious balance or when life is at stake, for instance during an infection or if we need to dissolve a sudden brain clot, but to believe we can maintain the balance of our complex system by drugs alone is a far fetched undertaking.

Until recently we have paid very little attention to the reversible nature of chronic illnesses. We are put on drugs, but we are seldom taken off them. This has left too many people on multiple drugs for life. Drugs are not harmless. Our casual use of medications is responsible for a staggering number of deaths attributed to prescription medications in the right dose and for the right condition. Drugs are best used with caution and whenever possible as a temporary measure until the body can regain a healthier balance.

Whole plant foods full of nutrients are non prescription drugs. By eating them every day we create a sustainable internal environment that moves us away from chronic inflammation and more toward health and wellness. Processed factory foods fortified with vitamins and minerals do not replace proper nutrition. The casual use of supplements is not supported by scientific research either for the prevention or protection against disease. What is more, an excess of vitamins, minerals, and other nutritional supplements taxes the liver and kidneys with the work of eliminating them, (not to mention the work of cleaning our public water supply). The only vitamin that all animals including humans need to consume is B_{12}. (More in the Micronutrient Section.)

If we avoid animal products it means we ingest less arachidonic acid from which to make chemicals such as inflammatory prostaglandins. Increasing plant foods from the extensively researched brassica family of vegetables (cruciferous) and which is mentioned throughout this book stimulates the body's production of enzymes that break down carcinogens and help maintain the integrity of the tumor suppressor p 53 protein, which monitors cell reproduction and DNA repair.

A diet of antioxidant rich foods including fruits, vegetables, legumes, and whole grains lowers the risk of disease. Even after years of abuse, a body treated to excellent nourishment will respond in kind. In the weeks and months after we eliminate oils, flour and sugar, meat and cheese, and replace them with whole plants, the body will slow down destruction and reverse as much disease as it can.

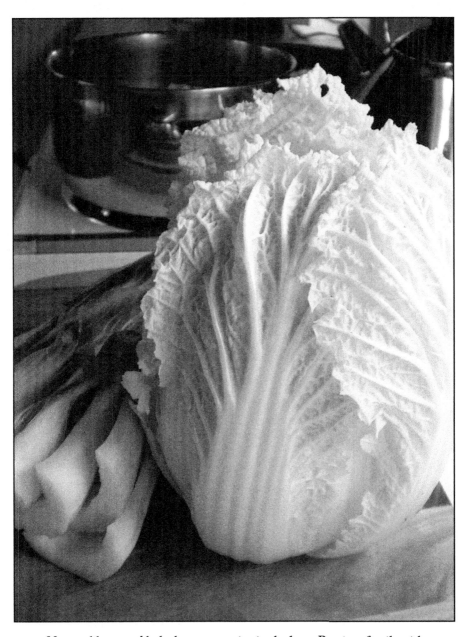

Napa cabbage and bok choy are cousins in the large Brasicca family with powerful nourishing benefits and delicate flavor.

"The human race has had long experience and a fine tradition in surviving adversity, but we now face a task for which we have little experience, the task of surviving prosperity."

—Alan Gregg 1890–1957, Rockefeller Foundation

Part V

Food in Medicine Around the World
and
Sustaining an Anti-inflammatory
Effect With Food

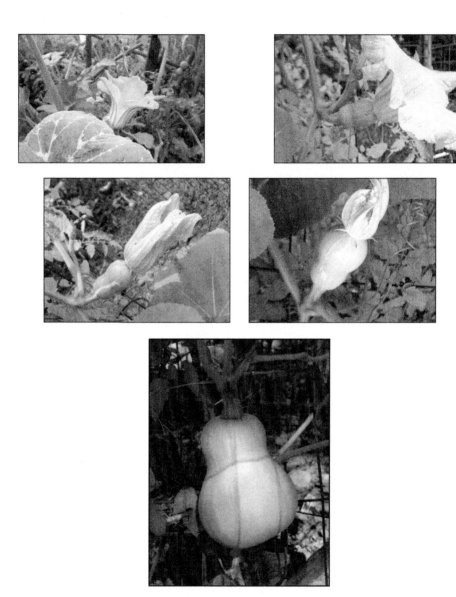

A few years ago seeds from a butternut squash that I had used in the kitchen
fell near the compost pile and grew a vine. Large flowers at the end of long
spindly stems fell off in two days. However, one grew on a shorter stem
and its base or ovary swelled and swelled reaching full squash size
in a few weeks with the flower still attached even as it shriveled.
The next time you hold a fruit in your hands you may discover
the remnants of petals on the end opposite its stem.

Sustaining an Anti-inflammatory Effect With Food

*T*his part summarizes diseases common in the United States, their prevalence in the world, mainstream treatment, and nutritional recommendations.

Diseases common to the US show extreme variability around the globe. This observation is not attributed to genetic differences, but to the food and lifestyle of modernized societies. A common effect of the western lifestyle characterized by excess food consumption, sedentary habits, and smoking, is chronic inflammation which in turn is associated with destruction of normal tissue.

Although nutrition counseling can improve an individual's health and save money on health-care costs, it is often not covered by insurance. The National Academy of Sciences' Institute of Medicine (IOM) deems nutritional therapy a cost effective component of medical therapy helping people manage conditions such as high-blood pressure, high cholesterol, kidney and heart problems, and diabetes. Even after a few sessions of nutritional counseling a person could lower cholesterol enough to the point of no longer needing cholesterol medication. According to the IOM report, nutrition therapy can mean a savings of millions of dollars. For example, if Medicare beneficiaries with high-blood pressure received nutrition therapy, healthcare costs could be cut by over 50 million dollars over a five-year period. Applied to every disease the cost savings could be staggering.

ACNE

PREVALENCE: Acne vulgaris is common among 50% of adolescents and adults in the United States. Among people who eat plant based diets acne is barely known, but when such people move to westernized countries and adopt the American diet, they develop rates of acne that match their new host country. These astonishing findings are common to most chronic illnesses and deserve our attention.

MEDICAL RX: Treatment based on the association between diet and acne continues to accumulate, but has been pushed aside in lieu of drugs. For more than three decades the success of acne treatment has been largely due to two topical drugs with strong anti-inflammatory properties: tretinoin and clindamycin.

NUTRITIONAL APPROACH: The insulin-like growth factor (IGF-1) normally present in milk (cow as well as human) is intended for growing infants, but cow's milk consumed later in life contributes to the formation of acne by stimulating sebaceous glands and the synthesis of androgens. A diet high in sugar and flour induces high levels of insulin and has a similar effect. Critical first steps in the prevention and treatment of acne include the elimination of dairy products, the reduction of foods high in flour and sugar, and a return to normal weight.

REFERENCES:
1. Cordain L, Lindeberg S, Hurtado M, Hill K, and Brand-Miler: Acne vulgaris: a disease of Western civilization. *J Arch Dermatol.* 2002 Dec;138(12):1584-90.
The researchers found no cases of acne among the Kitavan Islanders of Papua New Guinea or the Ache hunter gatherers of Paraguay. They postulate that the absence of acne cannot be attributed to genetics, but rather to environmental factors such as diet. Indeed, these populations eat a diet much less processed than Westernized counterparts.
2. Adebamowo CA, Spiegelman D, Danby FW, Frazier AL, Willett WC. Holmes MD: High school dietary dairy intake and teenage acne. *J Am Acad Dermatol.* 2005 Feb;52(2):207-14.
Abstract: The authors retrospectively examined data from 47,355 women who were part of the Nurses Health Study II. The women who had physician-diagnosed severe teenage acne in 1989 were asked in the year 1998 to complete questionnaires on high school diet. The purpose was to evaluate whether intakes of dairy foods during high school were associated with physician-diagnosed severe teenage acne. Taking into account age, age at menarche, body mass index, and energy intake, they found a positive association between acne and the intake of total milk and skim milk as well as instant breakfast drinks, sherbet, cottage cheese, and cream cheese.
3. Hogewoning AA et al: Prevalence and risk factors of inflammatory acne vulgaris in rural and urban Ghanaian schoolchildren. *British Journal of Dermatology.* 2009 161, pp 475-477.

The authors looked at prevalence of inflammatory acne vulgaris in Ghanaian schools and found that the incidence varied from as low as 1.3% in the rural areas to as high as 28.4% in the urban areas. It is likely that rural children in the study had limited access to processed products and refined carbohydrates, which might help explain the difference in acne prevalence between the two groups. The main factors associated with the increased risk of acne are: living in an urban area, increasing age, female gender, and high BMI.

4. Veith WB, Silverberg NB: The association of acne vulgaris with diet. *Cutis* 2011 Aug;88(2):84-91. There is a high association between acne and the high glycemic load of the Western diet, refined sugar products, the obesity epidemic, and certain dairy products. The data suggest that the casein component of whey is the most comedogenic. (The milk protein curdles separating into solids and liquid whey.)

ASTHMA, OTITIS, RHINITIS, SINUSITIS

PREVALENCE: Asthma has become a public health concern in affluent Western countries where 26 million people were suffering from this condition in 2010, an increase of 1% from the previous year. Being overweight or having a high BMI more than doubles the risk of this chronic inflammatory disease of the airways. Otitis, rhinitis, and sinusitis share some common triggers.

MEDICAL Rx: Corticosteroids, regarded the most potent anti-inflammatory agents available, suppress most of the inflammatory mediators involved in asthma except for leukotrienes. Leukotrienes increase mucus production and cause spasm and swelling of the airways. When corticosteroids are not enough, leukotriene inhibitors alter the production of these potent chemicals and prove useful.

NUTRITIONAL APPROACH: Plant linoleic acid → arachidonic acid → leukotriens. The human body uses plant Linoleic acid to make just the amount of arachidonic acid that it needs. Excess already made arachidonic acid found in animal products is used to produce leukotrienes. Eliminating animal products especially dairy lowers leukotriene production which could reduce or altogether eliminate the need for asthma medications.

REFERENCES:

1. Hong SJ, Lee MS, Lee SY, et al: High body mass index and dietary pattern are associated with childhood asthma. *Pediatr Pulmonol.* 2006 Dec;41(12):1118-24.

The results of this study from Korean elementary schoolchildren indicate that BMI may be an independent risk factor for the development of asthma symptoms in boys. A lower BMI which is associated with a diet of fresh seafood, fruit, and vegetables, may contribute to protect against the development of asthma symptoms.

2. Mohamed S Al-Hajjaj: Bronchial asthma in developing countries: A major social and economic burden. *Ann Thorac Med.* 2008 Apr-Jun; 3(2): 39–40.

The traditionally low incidence of bronchial asthma in developing countries is becoming a major health issue. This is a result of increased urbanization, more westernized diets, improved standard of living, decrease in exercise rates, more dust mites, and more pollution.

3. Nagel G, Weinmayr G, Kleiner A, García-Marcos L, Strachan DP: Effect of diet on asthma and allergic sensitisation in the International Study on Allergies and Asthma in Childhood (ISAAC) Phase Two. *Thorax.* 2010 Jun;65(6):516-22. doi: 10.1136/thx.2009.128256.

More frequent consumption of fruit, vegetables, and fish was associated with a lower lifetime prevalence of asthma, whereas high burger consumption was associated with higher lifetime asthma prevalence.

4. Allan K, Devereux G: Diet and asthma: nutrition implications from prevention to treatment. *J Am Diet Assoc* 2011 Feb;111(2):258-68. doi: 10.1016/j.jada.2010.10.048.

Observational studies report inverse associations between asthma and dietary antioxidants such as vitamin E, vitamin C, carotenoids, selenium, polyphenols, and fruit, as well as polyunsaturated fatty acids (PUFAs), and vitamin D. Noteworthy, supplementing the diets of adult asthmatics with antioxidants and omega-3 PUFAs has minimal or no clinical benefit, which continues to support two important notions: 1. Whole foods offer benefits beyond those of a supplement pill 2. A poor diet cannot be made better simply by adding supplements.

ALLERGIES AND ECZEMA

PREVALENCE: The Academy of Allergy, Asthma, and Immunology, reports that over the past fifty years there has been a rise in the prevalence of allergic disease in the industrialized world. Developing countries, such as Mexico, Chile, Kenya, Algeria, and countries in Southeast Asia, are also showing a rapid increase in cases of children's eczema. Since genetic factors could not change in such a short time, the reason for these unprecedented developments is believed to be environmental.

Atopic dermatitis or eczema: An itchy, inflammatory skin disorder which affects nearly 1 in 5 children living in developed countries. The vast majority show symptoms by the age of 5 years and more than half present before the age of 1 year. Although the cause is not fully understood, it seems clear that environmental, together with immune, genetic, metabolic, infectious, and neuroendocrine factors, all play a role.

Food allergy: Between 2% to 4% of adults and 5% to 10% of children are allergic to some food, most frequently: cow's milk, eggs, tree nuts, and peanuts. These allergic reactions can affect skin, gut, eyes, nose, and throat, and range from mild to moderate. A small subset of people react with life threatening anaphylaxis. Pharmaceutical drugs may be responsible for 20% of the severe reaction fatalities.

MEDICAL Rx: The mainstay of eczema treatment is a corticosteroid applied to the skin to block pro allergic cytokines and suppress inflammation. Two powerful non steroid medications have been added to the list: pimecrolimus and tacrolimus. These are from a class of drugs known as calcineurin and have impressive antitumor and immunosuppressive actions.

During allergic anaphylactic emergencies the goal is to prevent the airways from swelling shut. Patients with this type of reaction should stay away from the offending food and always carry emergency injectable epinephrine.

NUTRITIONAL APPROACH: There is a small fraction of children that have a documented food allergy; 90% are to cow's milk, peanuts, tree nuts (such as almonds, cashews, walnuts), eggs, fish (such as bass, cod, flounder), shellfish (such as crab, lobster, shrimp), soy, and wheat. The simple elimination of milk and eggs significantly improves more than 50% of children with atopic dermatitis. Since these foods are not essential, they all can be safely eliminated from the diet.

REFERENCE:
Scott H Sicherer, MD: Food for Thought on Prevention and Treatment of Atopic Disease Through Diet. *The Journaal of Pediatrics*. Oct 2007, Vol. 151, Issue 4, Pages 331-333.

AUTISM SPECTRUM DISORDER AND ADHD

PREVALENCE: The conditions lumped within this group have very heterogeneous manifestations.

MEDICAL Rx: Drug treatment is based on slowly and systematically addressing the various components and expressions of the disorder.

NUTRITIONAL APPROACH: The nutrients in whole plants cannot be replaced by supplements. Excellent whole food nutrition supplies the necessary macro and micronutrients essential for the brain to thrive.

REFERENCES:
Gordon Millichap and Michelle M. Yee: The Diet Factor in Attention-Deficit/Hyperactivity Disorder. *Pediatrics.* 2012;129:330–337. This article provides a comprehensive overview of the role of diet in the treatment of children with attention-deficit/ hyperactivity disorder (ADHD). While it intended to present diet as a last ditch effort when pharmacotherapy proved unsatisfactory or unacceptable it found something remarkable. In the Australian Raine study, a population based cohort of live births was followed to age 14 and the relationship between dietary patterns and ADHD was observed.[1] The "Western" dietary pattern which contains higher intakes of total fat, saturated fat, refined sugars, and sodium, deficient in omega-3 fatty acids, fiber, and folate, was associated with an ADHD diagnosis and also contributed to an increased tendency to obesity among non medicated ADHD children and adolescents. Conversly, the "Healthy" diet pattern, rich in fish, vegetables, fruit, legumes, and whole-grain foods, was not associated with ADHD diagnosis. [68] The article suggests that a relationship between a Western dietary pattern and ADHD may be mediated by other factors, such as poor family functioning and emotional distress leading to a craving for fat-rich snack foods. Whatever the specific cause, a modification of the child's dietary pattern may offer an alternative method of treatment of ADHD and less reliance on medications. Why not make an excellent diet the first and primary intervention?

NEURODEGENERATIVE DISORDERS: ALZHEIMER'S AND PARKINSON'S

PREVALENCE: Both of these are progressive neurodegenerative disorders. Alzheimer's affects 2% of the population of industrialized countries (an estimated 36 million people). Parkinson's is said to affect more than 4 million people worldwide with about 1 million identified in the United States alone.

MEDICAL Rx: In both conditions, neuroinflammation is out of control. The medical treatment is in evolution, however at least in Parkinson's the use of anti-inflammatory drugs appears to be a logical step.

NUTRITIONAL APPROACH: A naturally anti inflammatory low in fat plant based diet is an essential component of the treatment.

REFERENCES:

1. William B. Grant: Dietary Links to Alzheimer's Disease. *Alzheimer's Disease Review.* 2, 42-55, 1997.

There is strong evidence that the incidence and prevalence of Alzheimer's Disease (AD) is affected by diet. High risk factors include alcohol, fat, refined carbohydrates, salt, and high caloric consumption. Healthy diets should be considered the first line of defense against the development and progression of AD, as well as all other chronic degenerative diseases. The highest correlation for incidence and prevalence of AD was found in the 3-5 years before the study period, which suggests that diet modifications late in life can still affect the risk of developing AD. Exercise was found to reduce the incidence of stroke for men and should also reduce the risk of developing AD.

2. Mattson, MP: Gene-diet interactions in brain aging and neurodegenerative disorders. *Ann Intern Med.* 2003 Sep 2;139(5 Pt 2):441-4. Laboratory of Neurosciences, National Institute on Aging, Gerontology Research Center, Baltimore, MD 21224, USA.

Abstract: There are many examples of people who live one hundred or more years with little evidence of a decline in brain function. Many others are not so fortunate and develop a neurodegenerative disorder, such as Alzheimer disease or Parkinson disease. Although an increasing number of genetic factors that may affect risk are being identified, emerging findings suggest that dietary factors play major roles in determining whether the brain ages successfully or not. Dietary factors may interact with genes to either promote or prevent the degeneration of neurons. Epidemiologic findings suggest that high-calorie diets, folic acid deficiency, and elevated homocysteine levels may render the brain vulnerable to age-related neurodegenerative disorders, particularly in persons with a genetic predisposition.

3. Whitton PS: Neuroinflammation and the prospects for anti-inflammatory treatment of Parkinson's disease. *Curr Opin Investig Drugs.* 2010 Jul;11(7):788-94. The School of Pharmacy, Department of Pharmacology, London, UK.

4. William B. Grant: Trends in Diet and Alzheimer's Disease during the Nutrition Transition in Japan and Developing Countries. *Journal of Alzheimer's Disease.* Volume 38, Number 3, 2014 Pages 611-620.
Abstract: Alzheimer's disease (AD) rates in Japan and developing countries have risen rapidly in recent years. Researchers have associated factors such as the Western diet, obesity, alcohol consumption, and smoking with risk of AD. The authors of this study conclude that Alzheimer's Disease rates will continue to rise in non-Western countries unless we address major risk factors involving diet, obesity, and smoking.

OSTEOARTHRITIS

PREVALENCE: Osteoarthritis (OA) is the most common joint disorder around the world. Obesity is one of the strongest and best-established risk factors of OA. Being overweight or obese is associated with five to ten times the risk of osteoarthritis. Although weight bearing joints such as knees and hips are most commonly involved, the common involement of non weight bearing joints such as hands and wrists supports the role of circulating inflammatory cytokins in overweight and obese individuals. Osteoarthritis is not inherently due to growing older.

MEDICAL Rx: Analgesics, exercise, and weight reduction, all reduce pain.

NUTRITIONAL APPROACH: Weight loss reduces joint stress and lowers circulating inflammatory cytokins, making excellent nutrition the primary approach to osteoarthritis.

REFERENCE: Johns Hopkins Arthritis Center

RHEUMATOID ARTHRITIS

PREVALENCE: Rheumatoid arthritis (RA) is an autoimmune condition which in developing countries has lower prevalence and runs a milder course. The higher prevalence of RA seems to correlate with urbanization.

MEDICAL Rx: Targeted immune modulators, also referred as biologics, form a relatively new class of drugs used in the treatment of chronic inflammation and inappropriate immune response. Biologics work by selectively blocking steps in the inflammatory and immune cascades of diseases such as rheumatoid arthritis, psoriasis, ulcerative colitis, and inflammatory bowel disease.

RECENT HISTORY: The US Food and Drug Administration (FDA) has approved ten biologics: infliximab Remicade and etanercept Enbrel (1998), anakinra Kineret (2001), adalimumab Humira (2002), alefacept Amevive (2003), efalizumab (2003), abatacept Orencia (2005), rituximab Rituxan (2006), natalizumab Tysabri (2008), and certolizumab pegol Cimzia (2008). Plus golimumab Simponi, tocilizumab Actemra, and ustekinumab Stelara.

NUTRITIONAL APPROACH: There is significant evidence that plant based diets play a protective role against the signs and symptoms of rheumatoid arthritis. The elimination of animal products and other foods frequently implicated as allergens will improve many rheumatoid arthritis patients. Start by eliminating milk and eggs, peanuts, almonds, cashews, walnuts; bass, cod, flounder; shellfish such as crab, lobster, and shrimp; plus soy, and wheat.

REFERENCES:

1. I. Hafström, et al: A vegan diet free of gluten improves the signs and symptoms of rheumatoid arthritis: the effects of arthritis correlate with a reduction in antibodies to food antigens. *Rheumatology.* 2001;40:1175-1179. This is the first controlled study to demonstrate that a vegan diet exclusively from plants and free of gluten (wheat, rye, and barley) has long term beneficial effects on the signs and symptoms of RA.

2. Kalla AA, Tikly M, South Africa: Rheumatoid arthritis in the developing world. *Best Pract Res Clin Rheumatol.* 2003 Oct;17(5):863-75. The general impression is that rheumatoid arthritis has a lower prevalence and a milder course in developing countries. Epidemiological studies from different regions show that this is possibly related to absent or delayed urbanization.

3. Dorothy J. Pattison PhD[1], Deborah P. M. Symmons MD, et al: Dietary risk factors for the development of inflammatory polyarthritis: Evidence for a role of high level of red meat consumption. *Arthritis Rheum.* 2004;50:3804-3812. The results of this study demonstrate that a high level of red meat consumption is an independent risk factor for the development of inflammatory polyarthritis.

MULTIPLE SCLEROSIS

PREVALENCE: There are roughly 300,000 people suffering from Multiple Sclerosis (MS) in North America today and about 2,500,000 in the world. The incidence of MS and of other inflammatory autoimmune disorders is increasing pointing to nongenetic factors. It remains low in places such as Japan and some African countries where saurated fat intake is very low. Relatively recent changes in lifestyle, diet, and the use of antimicrobials, can create an altered balance in our resident biota (gastrointestinal microbial population) and appear to be associated with numerous diseases, including obesity, diabetes, rheumatoid arthritis, autism, and MS—where we find rogue immune activity throughout the body and brain.

MEDICAL R_X: Unsuccessful attempts to modulate the disease plus management of symptoms.

NUTRITION: The most consistent dietary association with MS is found in milk and dairy products. Eliminating this and other sources of satuated fat is associated with countless other benefits, such as reducing obesity and heart disease.

REFERENCES:
1. Kei E Fujimura, Nicole A Slusher, Michael D Cabana, and Susan V Lynch, PhD: Role of the gut microbiota in defining human health. *Expert Rev Anti Infect Ther*. 2010 Apr; 8(4).435-454.
2. Johannes Guggenmos, Anna S Schubart, Sherry Ogg, et al: Antibody cross-reactivity between myelin oligodendrocyte glycoprotein and the milk protein butyrophilin in multiple sclerosis. *The Journal of Immunology*. 02/2004; 172(1):661-668.

CANCERS

PREVALENCE: With the exception of esophagus, stomach, liver, and cervical, the rate of cancer is highest in developed countries. Cancer of the pancreas, prostate, and colon are many times more common in developed countries. According to the World Health Organization: while breast cancer is the top cancer in women (both in the developed and the developing world) the increasing incidence in the developing world is due to increased life expectancy, increased urbanization, and the adoption of western lifestyles.

MEDICAL Rx: Cancer can be diagnosed during any of its many stages: initiation, promotion, progression, and metastasis. The aim of cancer treatment, whether surgical, chemical, or radiation, is to reduce the load of cancer cells at that stage in order to give the body a chance to regain a healthier balance.

Especially during chemotherapy and radiation the organism's ability to defend itself is significantly curtailed, so attention to nutrition is essential in all phases of cancer treatment.

NUTRITION: Given the emerging role of animal protein in the initiation, promotion, progression, and metastasis of cancer, plant based diets are best not just for cancer protection but also during cancer treatment.

REFERENCES:
1. Alpha-Tocopherol Beta-Carotene (ATBC) cancer prevention trial. *N Engl J Med*. 1994;330(15):1029-1035.
This is a very publicized study from Finland. The important point of this study is that while foods rich in beta carotenes are known to protect smokers and non smokers against the development of lung cancer, they do not behave the same way when taken as supplements, where beta carotenes appeared to do the opposite and increased the risk of lung cancer.
2. Lawrence H. Kushi, Tim Byers, Colleen Doyle, Elisa V. Bandera, Marji McCullough, Ted Gansler, Kimberly S. Andrews, Michael J. Thun and The American Cancer Society 2006. Nutrition and Physical Activity Guidelines Advisory Committee for Cancer Prevention—Reducing the Risk of Cancer With Healthy Food Choices and Physical Activity. *CA Cancer J Clin* 2006;56;254-281.

CONSTIPATION

PREVALENCE: Constipation is one of the most common digestive complaints in the U.S. affecting almost 20% of the population. It is common among those who adopt a Western diet and less common in Asians. People eating diets low in plants and high in milk and cheese have intestinal content that cannot retain much water and moves too slowly, resulting in dry hard stools. In contrast, the stools of people who eat enough plants and plant fiber are like a sponge which drags waste in shorter time while holding on to water, resulting in frequent bowel movements easy to pass.

MEDICAL Rx: A conservative approach includes adding fiber to the diet so stools can retain water plus adding stimulants to accelerate gut motility. There are many remedies sold for constipation and they can be grouped in the following categories: 1. plant and other fibers that keep water in the stools; 2. stimulants that irritate the gut making it move; 3. drinking more water (which will keep stools moist only if there is enough fiber in the food or if the irritated bowels are moving faster than their ability to absorb the water that you drink—like when we have diarrhea); 4. then we start grasping at straws. For example: Magnesium supplement, which is sold as a remedy for constipation, is an abundant mineral in plants, which is what we should be consuming in the first place!

NUTRITION APPROACH: Constipation is treated (and most importantly prevented) by eliminating dairy products associated with slowing peristalsis (gut movement) and by increasing whole plant foods rich in fiber, which retain water and help intestinal motility.

REFERENCES:
1. GIacono, MD et al: Intolerance of Cow's Milk and Chronic Constipation in Children. *N Engl J Med.* 1998;339:1100-1104.
Intolerance of cow's milk can cause severe perianal lesions with pain on defecation and consequent constipation. In the children who remained off dairy for two weeks, sixty-eight percent responded with no more constipation. Incidentally, many of the children who responded favorably to the elimination of dairy were children who also suffered from higher frequency of coexistent rhinitis, dermatitis, or bronchospasm compared to those with no response. In other words, by eliminating cow's milk many other unsuspected conditions also improve.

GASTROESOPHAGEAL REFLUX (GERD)

PREVALENCE: GERD is the most common upper gastrointestinal disorder in developed countries. Acid reflux affects 30 million Americans (10% of the population), yet it is relatively rare in developing countries of Africa and Asia. Diets low in plant fiber are associated with the greatest risks for acid reflux. Symptoms which could include a burning sensation in the chest, a disagreeable taste in the mouth, and chronic cough, are exacerbated by fatty foods, alcohol, and smoking. The statistics for GERD around the globe follow obesity, which more than doubles the risk.

MEDICAL Rx: Proton pump inhibitors (PPIs) stop the secretion of stomach acid preventing the symptoms of acid burn but not the reflux itself. Bacteria are able to survive the acid free stomach and the persisting night time reflux is associated with higher incidence of aspiration pneumonia in adults. These drugs, with direct effect on neutrophils, monocytes, endothelial, and epithelial cells, have also been shown to have antioxidant properties—they modulate inflammation, reduce oxidative stress, and help repair mucosal injury in the small intestine. PPIs appear to influence a variety of inflammatory disorders both within and outside of the gastrointestinal tract.

NUTRITIONAL APPROACH: A plant based diet low in fat and processed foods will help reduce GERD. Importantly and for long term benefit: avoid overeating and return to normal weight.

REFERENCES:
1. Mehdi Saberi-Firoozi, Farnaz Khademolhosseini, Maryam Yousefi, Davood Mehrabani, Najaf Zare, Seyed Taghi Heydari: Risk factors of gastroesophageal reflux disease in Shiraz, southern Iran. *World J Gastroenterol.* 2007 November 7;13(41): 5486-5491.
Although the effect of lifestyle on GERD has not been firmly elucidated, this study suggests that diets high in fat are implicated in the symptoms of acid reflux.

1. Mehdi Saberi-Firoozi, Farnaz Khademolhosseini, Maryam Yousefi, Davood Mehrabani, Najaf Zare, Seyed Taghi Heydari: Risk factors of gastroesophageal reflux disease in Shiraz, southern Iran. *World J Gastroenterol.* 2007 November 7;13(41): 5486-5491.
In this cross sectional study, high dietary fat intake was associated with an increased risk of GERD symptoms and erosive esophagitis while high fibre intake correlated with a reduced risk of GERD symptoms.

INFLAMMATORY BOWEL DISEASE AND ULCERATIVE COLITIS

PREVALENCE: The incidence and prevalence of these conditions in western countries has been increasing over the past 50 years. Around 1 million people in the U.S. have some form of inflammatory bowel disease. Migrants from a low-risk region who move to a high-risk region match the risk of developing the disease within one generation.

MEDICAL Rx: Medications used to treat inflammatory bowel disease suppress the immune system and reduce inflammation.

NUTRITIONAL APPROACH: We must begin by mentioning that western dietary patterns with their high animal protein, processed flour and sugar, and low fiber content, increase the risk of inflammatory bowel disease by two to four times compared to those who avoid it and rely instead on plant based diets.

REFERENCES:
1. Silvio Danese, MD, and Claudio Fiocchi, MD: Ulcerative Colitis (and Crohn's disease). *N Engl J Med.* 2011; 365:1713-1725 November 3, 2011. Ulcerative colitis and Crohn's disease are disorders of modern society and their frequency in developed countries has been increasing since the mid-20th century. The westernized lifestyle of: smoking, diets high in fat and sugar, medication use, stress, and high socioeconomic status, are linked to the appearance of inflammatory bowel disease.

CELIAC DISEASE

PREVALENCE: This inflammatory disease affects less than 1% of the population of the United States. Its prevalence is the same in Europe and probably the world. People genetically predisposed react to the ingestion of gluten protein (found in wheat, rye, and barley) with varying degrees of damage to the lining of their small intestine.

MEDICAL Rx: Total avoidance of gluten for life.

NUTRITIONAL APPROACH: A plant centered diet (free from the gluten simply by avoiding wheat, rye, or barley) provides perfectly adequate nutrition for people with or without celiac disease. The person who insists on using processed foods for her gluten free diet will be forever reading labels. Since processed foods lack many components of excellent nutrition, such person is likely to also develop untold nutritional deficiencies.

REFERENCES:
1. Michelle Pietzac, MD: Celiac Disease, Wheat Allergy, and Gluten Sensitivity—when gluten free is not a fad. *J Parenter Enteral Nutr.* January 2012 vol. 36 no. 1 suppl 68S-75S.
As the gluten-free diet (GFD) gains in popularity with the general public, health practitioners are beginning to question its real health benefits. For those patients with celiac disease (CD), the GFD is medical nutrition therapy and the only proven treatment which improves symptoms and heals small bowel histology. Those with wheat allergy also benefit from the GFD, although these patients often do not need to restrict rye, barley, and oats from

their diet. The third category—gluten sensitivity—is a controversial subject. These patients have neither CD nor wheat allergy, but have varying degrees of symptomatic improvement on the GFD. Conditions in this category include dermatitis herpetiformis (DH), irritable bowel syndrome (IBS), and neurologic diseases such as gluten-sensitive ataxia and autism. It is important for patients and healthcare practitioners to understand the differences between these conditions, even though they may all respond to a GFD. Patients with CD can experience co-morbid nutrition deficiencies and are at higher risk for the development of cancers and other autoimmune conditions. Those with wheat allergy and gluten sensitivity are thought not to be at higher risk for these complications. Defining the symptoms and biochemical markers for gluten-sensitive conditions is an important area for future investigations and high-quality, large-scale randomized trials are needed to prove the true benefits of the GFD in this evolving field.

2. Alessio Fasano: Leaky Gut and Autoimmune Diseases. *Clinic Rev Allerg Immunol.* 2011 DOI 10.1007/s12016-011-8291-x; Mucosal Biology Research Center, University of Maryland School of Medicine.

The intercellular tight junctions (TJ) in the intestinal epithelial barrier together with the gut-associated lymphoid tissue and the neuroendocrine network control the equilibrium between tolerance and immunity to non-self antigens.

3. A Fasano: Zonulin and its regulation of intestinal barrier function: the biological door to inflammation, autoimmunity, and cancer. *Physiol Rev.* 2011 Jan;91(1):151-75. doi: 10.1152/physrev.00003.2008.

Abstract: The primary functions of the gastrointestinal tract have traditionally been perceived to be limited to the digestion and absorption of nutrients and to electrolytes and water homeostasis. A more attentive analysis of the anatomic and functional arrangement of the gastrointestinal tract, however, suggests that another extremely important function of this organ is its ability to regulate the trafficking of macromolecules between the environment and the host through a barrier mechanism. Together with the gut-associated lymphoid tissue and the neuroendocrine network, the intestinal epithelial barrier, with its intercellular tight junctions, controls the equilibrium between tolerance and immunity to non-self antigens. Zonulin is the only physiological modulator of intercellular tight junctions described so far that is involved in trafficking of macromolecules and therefore, in tolerance/immune response balance. When the finely tuned zonulin pathway is deregulated in genetically susceptible individuals, both intestinal and extraintestinal autoimmune, inflammatory, and neoplastic disorders can occur. This new paradigm subverts traditional theories underlying the development of these diseases and suggests that these processes can be arrested if the triggers that interplay between genes and environmental is prevented by reestablishing the zonulin-dependent intestinal barrier function. This review is timely given the increased interest in the role of a "leaky gut" in the pathogenesis of several pathological conditions targeting both the intestine and extraintestinal organs.

DIVERTICULAR DISEASE

PREVALENCE: There are few diseases whose incidence varies so much throughout the world as diverticulosis. Diverticula are weak out-pouches in the colon wall caused by increased pressure within the large intestine usually from chronic constipation; they are prone to infection and bleeding. Some Western nations have prevalence rates that approach 40% of the population. For example, by age 60 nearly half of Americans have diverticula. Developing countries in Asia and Africa have a prevalence well below that. However, as they assume a more Western lifestyle, especially a low–fiber diet and a sedentary lifestyle, they are showing increased rates of diverticulosis. The wide variation (from nil to nearly 30% of the population) is closely related to economic development.

MEDICAL Rx: The approach to diverticula found on routine colonoscopy or other imaging test is with a plant rich diet to correct constipation and improve the health of colon cells. Acute complications like inflammation or bleeding need immediate medical or surgical interventions. During the acute episode the bowel needs rest, which often means a temporary low fiber diet. Once recovered, the diet should consist of whole plant foods high in fiber including fruits, legumes, grains, vegetables, nuts, and seeds.

NUTRITIONAL APPROACH: Diets high in red meat and total fat, which are also low in dietary fiber, correlate with diverticular disease. Vegetarians, whose diets tend to be higher in fiber compared to non vegetarians, have a very low incidence of diverticular disease.

REFERENCES:
1. S Prasad, MPH, B Ewingman, MD: Let them eat nuts—this snack is safe for diverticulosis patients. *Journal of Family Practice.* February 2009, Vol. 58, No. 2: 82-84.
Nuts have many health benefits and we know of no reason for patients with diverticulosis to avoid them.

DYSMENORRHEA

PREVALENCE: Almost 50% of women younger than 30 experience moderate to severe pain during menstruation.

MEDICAL Rx: Women with dysmenorrhea have been shown to produce 7 times more prostaglandin F2 alpha than women without dysmenorrhea. When the prostaglandin F2 alpha (a strong pro inflammatory chemical) is released at high levels into the bloodstream it causes the uterus to spasm sometimes leaving it painfully without blood supply like when the heart feels angina pain. The mainstay approach has been prompt anti inflammatory drugs used on the first day of menstruation.

NUTRITION APPROACH: Vegetarian, low-fat, non dairy diets have helped many women reduce the symptoms of painful menstrual cramps.

REFERENCES:
1. Linda French, MD: Dysmenorrhea Am Fam Physician. 2005 Jan 15;71(2):285-291.
Few studies have examined the effect of lifestyle-modification interventions in the management of dysmenorrhea. One cross-over study, of low-fat vegetarian diet versus placebo pill, showed decreased duration and intensity of dysmenorrhea among women in the intervention group.
2. Mahkam Tavallaee, MD, Shahid Beheshti University: Prevalence of Menstrual Pain and Associated Risk Factors Among Iranian Women Research Project 2009. Simon Frazer University, Burnaby, BC, Canada.
Low fat diet and daily high consumption of fruits and vegetables correlates with lower levels of pain during menstruation. A high fiber diet leads to better elimination of estrogen in the feces. Vegetarian diets are associated with lower BMI, higher Sex Hormone Binding Globulin (SHBG), and lower circulating estrogen. Among other favorable conditions this causes reduced endometrium proliferation, lower levels of prostaglandins, and less myometrial contractions.

POLYCYSTIC OVARIAN SYNDROME (PCOS)

PREVALENCE: Polycystic ovarian syndrome (PCOS) is a common complex metabolic, endocrine, and reproductive disorder, affecting 4-8% of reproductive age women in developed countries. The core problem in up to 70% of women with this disorder seems to be resistance to insulin. Similar to diabetes, the prevalence of PCOS is on the rise in nations undergoing rapid nutritional transitions to Westernized diets and lifestyle. The manifestations of PCOS often include a cluster of conditions also known as metabolic syndrome: obesity especially around the waist, abnormal lipids, hypertension, and type 2 diabetes. Due to arterial endothelial dysfunction and a chronic low-grade inflammatory state, women with PCOS show increased risk of developing heart disease.

MEDICAL Rx: Since a fundamental problem in PCOS is insulin resistance, the first and most important step is weight loss and exercise—both of which improve sensitivity to insulin.

NUTRITIONAL APPROACH: A diet of whole grains (not refined), along with vegetables, legumes, and fruits, is low in fat and high in fiber. This not only improves weight but also helps reestablish the upset sex hormone balance.

REFERENCES:
Pier Giorgio Crosignani, et al: Overweight and obese anovulatory patients with polycystic ovaries: parallel improvements in anthropometric indices, ovarian physiology and fertility rate induced by diet. _Oxford Journals Medicine & Health Human Reproduction._ Volume 18, Issue 9, pp 1928-1932.

STONES: GALLSTONES / KIDNEY STONES / GOUT

PREVALENCE: Gallstones occur in about 10 to 20% of adults in developed countries. In fact, by age 75 about 35% of women and 20% of men have developed gallstones. The main risk factors seem to be an excess of animal protein and fat together with a lack of plant fiber. Obese people have double the risk than those of normal weight.

Kidney stones too, are common in developed countries. Almost 10% of Americans report a symptomatic stone once in their lifetime with a recurrence rate of over 50%. Diets high in animal protein, sodium, and colas, increase the risk of kidney stones.

In gout, urate crystals precipitate in joints and soft tissues causing great inflammation, damage, and pain. Being overweight and obese almost triples the risk. People who eat more red meat, poultry, or fish have significantly higher risk compared to those eating the least. While some studies show the consumption of dairy to be protective because it promotes the elimination of uric acid, its association with serious diseases such as prostate cancer and Parkinson's, makes this a dubious approach.

MEDICAL Rx: Symptomatic gallstones are treated by surgically removing the gall bladder. Symptomatic kidney stones are treated by surgically removing them through the urethra. Gout is treated with anti inflammatory drugs plus drugs to alter uric acid production and excretion.

NUTRITION APPROACH: A plant based diet eliminates most risk factors for all of these conditions—naturally high in fiber, low in fat, low in sodium, has no refined carbohydrates, and definitely meets our protein needs without exceeding them.

The gallstones in Western countries are composed mainly of cholesterol and are considered a direct result of the the diet of modern societies. A vegetarian diet and high fluid intake protect the majority of recurrent kidney stone-formers. Research continues to show that dietary consumption of meat and seafood is associated with an increased risk of gout.

REFERENCES:
1. Ada Cuevas MD, Juan Francisco Miguel MD, Silvana Zanlugo, PhD, and Flavio Nervi, MD: Diet as a Risk Factor for Cholesterol Gallstone Disease. *Journal of the American College of Nutrition*. Vol. 23, No. 3, 187–196 (2004).
2. Professor Monica Acalovschi: Cholesterol gallstones: from epidemiology to prevention. *Postgrad Med J.* 2001; 77:221-229 doi:10.1136/bmj.77.906.221. Descriptive epidemiology suggests consistently that the environmental factors which characterize modern Western civilization and urbanization may be responsible for most cholesterol rich gallstones. All these factors are amenable to prevention.
3. Chung, Jyi Tsai et al: Dietary Protein and the Risk of Cholecystectomy in a Cohort of US Women; The Nurses' Health Study. *Am. J. Epidemiol.* (2004) 160 (1): 11-18. The results suggest that increased consumption of vegetable protein (within an energy-balanced diet) can reduce the risk of cholecystectomy in women.
4. Charlotte H Dawson and Charles RV Tomson: Kidney stone disease: pathophysiology, investigation and medical treatment. *Clin Med.* October 1, 2012 vol. 12 no. 5 467-471.
5. Yuqing Zhang, et al: Purine-rich foods intake and recurrent gout attacks. *Ann Rheum Dis.* 2012;71:1448-1453 doi:10.1136/annrheumdis-2011-201215. "The study findings suggest that acute purine intake increases the risk of recurrent gout attacks by almost fivefold among gout patients. Avoiding or reducing amount of purine-rich foods intake, especially of animal origin, may help reduce the risk of gout attacks."

6. Hossam El Zawawy, MD, Brian F Mandell, MD, PhD: Managing gout: How is it different in patients with chronic kidney disease? *Cleveland Clinic Journal of Medicine.* December 2010 vol. 77 12 919-928. Altering the diet: Traditional advice confirmed - "The Health Professionals Follow-up Study prospectively examined the relation between diet and gout over 12 years in 47,150 men. The study confirmed some long-standing beliefs, such as that consuming meat, seafood, beer, and liquor increases the risk. Other risk factors were consumption of sugar-sweetened soft drinks and fructose, adiposity, weight gain, hypertension, and diuretic use. On the other hand, protein, wine, and purine-rich vegetables were not associated with gout flares. Low-fat dairy products may have a protective effect. Weight loss was found to be protective."

HEART DISEASE AND ITS RISK FACTORS

PREVALENCE: Each year almost 800,000 Americans have their first heart attack and another 500,000 have a second or third. Heart disease is associated with higher body mass index, high blood pressure, high fasting blood lipids, and diabetes. Surveys show that developing countries with lower levels of blood cholesterol, blood pressure, and body mass index have lower incidence of heart disease. Erectile dysfunction (also known as impotence), peripheral artery disease (characterized by intermittent pain in the legs with exercise) and coronary angina (which often presents with chest pain on exertion) are also manifestations of heart disease.

MEDICAL Rx: Many drugs are used to reduce heart disease symptoms and some risks. Surgical interventions are reserved for high risk patients with prominent symptoms. Although diet and lifestyle are the cornerstone of treatment, counseling patients on their importance and how to accomplish this remains suboptimal.

NUTRITION APPROACH: Diet regulates blood lipids, improves elasticity of the blood vessels (endothelial function), and lowers inflammation. Diet can slow down damage, arrest progression, and even regress disease. Given that the development of heart disease starts early in life, a protective diet ought to be standard practice from childhood.

REFERENCES:
1. Heart Disease: Exporting failure? Coronary heart disease and stroke in developing countries Heart Disease. *Int. J. Epidemiol.* (2001) 30 (2): 201-205. doi: 10.1093/ije/30.2.201.

2. Harpal S Buttar, DVM , Phd, Timao Li, PhD, and Nivedita Ravi, BSc: Clinical Cardiology: Prevention of cardiovascular diseases: Role of exercise, dietary interventions, obesity and smoking cessation. Exp Clin Cardiol. 2005 Winter; 10(4): 229–249. PMCID: PMC2716237.
3. K Srinath Reddy, MD, DM; Salim Yusuf, DPhil: Emerging Epidemic of Cardiovascular Disease in Developing Countries. Circulation. Current Perspectives 1998.
A cross-sectional survey of urban Delhi and its rural environs revealed that a higher prevalence of coronary heart disease in the urban sample was associated with higher levels of body mass index, blood pressure, fasting blood lipids (total cholesterol, ratio of cholesterol to HDL cholesterol, triglycerides), and diabetes. In addition, the increasing use of tobacco in many developing countries will also translate into higher mortality rates of cardiovascular, lung cancer, and other tobacco-related diseases.
4. Esselstyn, MD, Caldwell: Prevent and Reverse Heart Disease, Avery 2007.

SEXUAL DYSFUNCTION (formerly known as impotence)

During male excitation the penis arteries normally dilate and compress their partner veins acting like a tourniquet. The subsequent pooling of blood in the shaft causes an erection. If the arteries cannot produce nitric oxide they don't dilate, so blood pumped into the corpora cavernosa (shaft) returns through the veins just as quickly as it was pumped in and the penis remains flaccid.

In women, sexual function correlates better with psychological factors than with blood flow to the genital area and it appears that adequate blood flow or engorgement will often be ignored unless other propitious conditions are present.

PREVALENCE: Almost 10% of men in the U.S. have erectile dysfunction which is an early sign of heart disease. The risk of erectile dysfunction is greatly increased by obesity which in itself is associated with stiff arteries, elevated blood pressure, and poor circulation to every organ.

MEDICAL Rx: Nitric oxide gas is normally produced in the walls of blood vessels keeping them elastic. Drugs that donate nitric oxide (such as sildenafil - Viagra, and tadalafil - Cialis) impart temporary elasticity to the arteries by producing artificially high nitric oxide levels. Nitroglycerin is another such drug used to dilate coronary arteries and increase circulation to the heart. Drugs like sildenafil and tadalafil are used to dilate the penile arteries.

NUTRITIONAL APPROACH: A whole plant diet low in fat, paired with smoking cessation and exercise, will improve erectile function and immediately start reducing all cardiovascular risk factors.

REFERENCES:
1. Gupta, Murad, et al: The effect of lifestyle modification and cardiovascular risk factor reduction on erectile dysfunction: a systematic review and meta-analysis *Arch Intern Med.* 2011 Nov 14;171(20):1797-803. doi: 10.1001/archinternmed.2011.440. Epub 2011 Sep 12.
2. Basson, Rosemary MB, BS, MRCP: Female Sexual Response: The Role of Drugs in the Management of Sexual Dysfunction. *Obstetrics & Gynecology.* August 2001, Volume 98, Issue 2, p 350-353.

DIABETES AND INSULIN RESISTANCE

PREVALENCE: Type 2 diabetes represents 90% of all diabetes. About 90% of type 2 diabetes, which is rapidly becoming a worldwide pandemic, can be attributed to excess weight. People who grow largest around the waist (apple shaped obesity) develop persistent inflammation with increased risk for diabetes and heart disease. Additionally 197 million people worldwide have impaired glucose tolerance, which means they are incubating diabetes. By 2025 this number is expected to increase to 420 million.

Populations which have undergone westernization and urbanization (such as Arab, migrant Asian, Indian, Chinese, and the Hispanic communities in the U.S.) are at higher risk. Urban areas of the developing world have a prevalence of diabetes ranging from 14 to 20%. In contrast, population-based surveys of 75 communities in 32 countries show that where they have preserved a traditional more plant based lifestyle diabetes is rare.

Type 1 diabetes affects about 3 million Americans. For reasons still not entirely clear, the pancreas stops producing insulin and the person depends on daily insulin injections for life. Without insulin glucose accumulates to very high levels in the blood. The results are dehydration and severe chemical imbalances which could lead to coma and death. A low fat plant based diet helps to keep the insulin receptors functioning well (insulin sensitive) in both types of diabetes.

Type 2 diabetes affects close to 300 million people worldwide and over 20 million in the U.S. alone. During the early stages of this diabetes there is enough insulin, but saturated fat in the diet and deposits of fat inside the liver and other abdominal organs provoke a condition known as insulin resistance which keeps glucose from entering the cells.

The situation can devolve into the following cascade of metabolic derangements:

1. High glucose concentrations in the eyes which cause blurred vision.
2. High levels of glucose which are toxic to cells throughout the body and the brain.
3. Glucose spills in the urine dragging water out of the body, so tissues get dehydrated.
4. Glucose cannot enter the cells to be used for energy, so the person becomes weak and fatigued.
5. Fat and muscle are burned for fuel (instead of glucose) and the person unintentionally loses weight.
6. Eventually the exhausted pancreas cannot produce any more insulin, making one dependent on insulin injections.

MEDICAL Rx: A growing number of drugs help control diabetes. Metformin may have a role in reducing obesity-associated inflammation. Various other medications for diabetes either reduce insulin resistance or increase insulin production. Injected insulin adds itself to the insulin produced in the body, but without a balanced diet this often leads to weight gain which exacerbates the condition.

NUTRITIONAL APPROACH: A low fat plant based diet improves insulin sensitivity and can reverse Type 2 diabetes. It also reduces other risk factors which are associated with diabetes, like heart disease.

REFERENCES:
1. Brownlee, M: Biochemistry and molecular cell biology of diabetic complications. *Nature*, 2001 Dec 13;414(6865):813-20.
Patients who maintain high glucose levels in the blood have increased production of free radicals. These reactive oxygen species (ROS) damage the thin lining of blood vessels and activate inflammation. Within the fatty abdomen, this type of blood vessel injury further exacerbates local and generalized inflammation. When the insulin producing beta cell islets of the pancreas live in this inflammatory environment (characterized by cytokines, apoptotic

cells, immune cell infiltration, and amyloid deposits) they eventually die and are replaced with scar tissue. This inflammation is probably the combined consequence of high fat (hyperlipidemia), high sugar (hyperglycemia), and increased adipokines (which are secreted by fatty tissue and modulate the immune system).

2. Kitt Falk Petersen, and Gerald I. Shulman, Department of Internal Medicine, Department of Cellular & Molecular Physiology & Howard Hughes Medical Institute, Yale University School of Medicine, New Haven, Connecticut: New Insights into the Pathogenesis of Insulin Resistance in Humans Using Magnetic Resonance Spectroscopy. *Obesity*. 14:34S-40S (2006) © 2006 The North American Association for the Study of Obesity.

a. The primary cause of type 2 diabetes is unknown, however cross-sectional studies show insulin resistance in virtually all such patients, underscoring that insulin resistance plays a major role.

b. Prospective studies identify insulin resistance one to two decades before the onset of the disease. In fact insulin resistance in asymptomatic offspring of parents with type 2 diabetes is the best predictor for the later development of the disease.

c. Finally and most importantly, reducing insulin resistance prevents the development of diabetes.

3. Parvez Hossain, MD, Bisher Kawar, MD, and Meguid El Nahas, MD, PhD: Obesity and Diabetes in the Developing World - A Growing Challenge. *N Engl J Med* 2007; 356:213-215 January 18, 2007, DOI: 10.1056/NEJMp068177.

4. Barnard, MD, Neal: Program for Reversing Diabetes, Rodale 2008.

By 2007, more than 1 billion adults worldwide were overweight and more than 300 million were obese. According to the International Obesity Task Force at least 155 million children worldwide are overweight or obese. About 90% of type 2 diabetes is attributable to excess weight and about 18 million people die every year from cardiovascular disease, which is predisposed by diabetes and hypertension.

HYPERLIPIDEMIA

PREVALENCE: 70 million Americans have high cholesterol and 100 million have high triglycerides. High blood levels of these lipids are associated with heart disease.

MEDICAL Rx: The medical treatment of hyperlipidemia consists of diet and lifestyle changes. Statins, used to lower blood lipids, have a direct anti-inflammatory effect through inhibition of pro inflammatory cytokine and chemokine secretion, as well as the expression of adhesion molecule-1 on leukocytes. Statins are also potent modulators of endothelial nitric oxide synthase and have been shown to up-regulate nitric oxide (NO) production which helps to keep arteries elastic. On the down side, the long term use of these drugs is been studied for their potential association with increased risk of diabetes and cancer.

NUTRITIONAL APPROACH: The treatment of hyperlipidemia consists of diet and lifestyle changes. Hyperlipidemia is not considered refractory (resistant) until one has excluded all animal products and vegetable oils from the diet. Since high lipids are often seen in overweight patients, a whole plant based diet is the most effective.

> REFERENCE:
> Stone NJ, et al: Lifestyle as the Foundation for ASCVD Risk Reduction Efforts. *2013 ACC/AHA Blood Cholesterol Guideline.* Page 13, 2.1.
> It must be emphasized that adhering to a heart healthy diet, regular exercise habits, avoidance of tobacco products, and maintenance of a healthy weight remain critical components of health promotion and (Atherosclerotic and Cardiovascular Disease) ASCVD risk reduction, both prior to and in concert with the use of cholesterol-lowering drug therapies.

HYPERTENSION

PREVALENCE: One billion people have hypertension worldwide, 65 million in the U.S. alone. The key risk factors are a high fat and salt diet, being overweight or obese, excess alcohol consumption, and a sedentary lifestyle. Rarely some medications or other disorders could cause elevated blood pressure.

MEDICAL Rx: An array of prescription medications are used to control, not cure, hypertension.

NUTRITION APPROACH: The cure for hypertension is achieved by limiting alcohol, a return to normal weight, eating a low fat plant based diet naturally low in salt, and smoking cessation to avoid complications.

REFERENCE:
1. A Global Brief on Hypertension – World Health Organization 2013.
2. Yokoyama Y, Nishimura K, Barnard ND, Takegami M, Watanabi M, Sekikawa A, Okamura T, Miyamoto Y: Vegetarian diets and blood pressure: a meta-analysis. *JAMA Intern Med.* 2014 Apr;174(4):577-87. Conclusions and Relevance: Consumption of vegetarian diets is associated with lower BP. Such diets could be a useful nonpharmacologic means for reducing BP.

INSOMNIA

PREVALENCE: Sleep deprivation has serious consequences—irritability, increased appetite, lack of focus and concentration, depression and anxiety, aches and pains, not to mention accidents and car crashes. It is estimated that 10% of the world's population suffers with insomnia, which is broadly defined as having trouble falling or staying asleep. Although sleep is a natural occurring event in human life (we fall asleep when we are tired and wake up rested), we override this natural phenomenon in a variety of ways. For example: many people living sedentary lifestyles are not physically tired at the end of the day. Others have such inconsistent work schedules that they never establish a predictable sleep pattern. Being overweight or obese can be associated with sleep disruption through sleep apnea or acid reflux, both of which have become ubiquitous. Stress is associated with anxious or depressed thoughts that can interfere with sleep. Using some prescription medications, sedative drugs, alcohol, maintaining an inconsistent or disruptive routine, taking stimulants such as caffeine, or eating before going to bed, can all interfere with natural sleep. Although a small percentage of people report disrupted sleep with none of the above, the majority can address their sleeplessness by removing obstacles from sleep's way rather that by trying to induce it artificially.

MEDICAL Rx: Treatment should include addressing any underlying conditions, such as obesity and sleep apnea plus logical suggestions such as sleep hygiene routines, daytime exercise, and no TV in the bedroom. If short term medications are used they should always include a plan for recovering a healthier sleep-wake cycle.

NUTRITION APPROACH: There are no particular foods to cure insomnia, but being well nourished is the foundation to the body's excellent function.

REFERENCE:
Sleep Foundation Organization: http://sleepfoundation.org/sleep-topics/
diet-exercise-and-sleep/page/0%2C3/.

MOOD DISORDERS/ DEPRESSION AND OTHERS

PREVALENCE: According to a study supported by WHO: in any community almost 5% of the residents have suffered from depression in the last year. The World Health Organization (WHO) announced in 2010 that at least 350 million people suffer from depression worldwide. In depression, there are limited concentrations of circulating T lymphocytes and other immune cells which perform a variety of "housekeeping" tasks and carry out essential immunosurveillance in the central nervous system (CNS).

MEDICAL Rx: A variety of drugs try to address the biochemical imbalances observed in mood disorders.

NUTRITIONAL APPROACH: People whose diets consist of processed meats, chocolates, sweets, fried foods, refined cereals, and high-fat dairy products, are more likely to report symptoms of depression. A diet of whole plant foods composed of 70% carbohydrate and 10% protein protects against obesity, diabetes, and also against depression.

REFERENCES:
1. Almudena Sánchez-Villegas, Estefania Toledo, Jokin de Irala, Miguel Ruiz-Canela, Jorge Pla-Vidal and Miguel A Martínez-González: Fast-food and commercial baked goods consumption and the risk of depression. *Public health Nutrition/* Volume 15 / Issue 03 / March 2012, pp 424-432. In 493 cases reported, the consumption of fast food (such as hamburgers, sausages, pizza) plus commercial baked goods and processed pastries (such as muffins, doughnuts, croissants) was associated with a higher risk of depression.
2. Bradley M. Appelhans, PhD, Matthew C. Whited, PhD, Kristin L. Schneider, PhD, Yunsheng Ma, PhD, MD, MPH, Jessica L. Oleski, MA, Philip A. Merriam, MSPH, Molly E. Waring, PhD, Barbara C. Olendzki, RD, MPH, Devin M. Mann, MD, MS, Ira S. Ockene, MD, Sherry L. Pagoto, PhD: Depression Severity, Diet Quality, and Physical Activity in Women with Obesity and Depression. *Journal of the Academy of Nutrition and Dietetics* Volume 112, Issue 5, Pages 693–698, May 2012.

Associations with diet were primarily driven by greater intake of sugar, saturated fat, and sodium. Among treatment-seeking women with major depressive disorder (MDD) and obesity, more severe depression was associated with poorer overall diet quality, but not physical activity.

OBESITY

PREVALENCE: The International Obesity Taskforce (2010) estimates that approximately 1.0 billion adults are overweight (BMI 25-29.9) and an additional 475 million are obese (BMI over 30) worldwide. In the United States, more that a third of adult men and women are obese. The statistics are similar for children. Obesity is associated with numerous co-morbidities including an increased risk for coronary heart disease, type 2 diabetes, gallstones, cancers, and disability.

MEDICAL Rx: Drug treatments have been woefully ineffective often doing more harm than good. Bariatric surgeries have demonstrated short term success, with most patients gaining their weight back within three years. Healthful changes in diet and lifestyle remain the cornerstone of the treatment of obesity, however given the sparse nutrition education among physicians and the lack of adequate counsel given to patients, at the present this does not hold promise. This book attempts to make a difference.

NUTRITION APPROACH: When a person has reached overweight and obese proportions, any method can be used to get weight loss started, but long lasting benefits are achieved only with fundamental changes in food consumption and lifestyle. This most logical approach offers a sure way to reverse the obesity epidemic. It is difficult in a society that fuels weight gain, but not impossible.

REFERENCES:
1. Bulletin of the World Health Organization Print version ISSN 0042-9686 *Bull World Health Organ* vol.82 n.12 Genebra Dec. 2004.
A landmark review of studies on socioeconomic status (SES) and obesity was published before 1989 and supported the view that obesity in the developing world would turn out to be essentially a disease of the socioeconomic elite. However, the present review on studies conducted in adult populations from developing countries, published between 1989 and 2003, shows a different

relationship between SES and obesity. The following three main conclusions emerge:

a. Obesity in the developing world can no longer be considered a disease of groups with higher SES.

b. As the country's gross national product (GNP) increases, the burden of obesity in each developing country tends to shift towards groups with lower SES.

c. The shift of obesity in favor of women with low SES apparently occurs at an earlier stage of economic development than it does for men.

2. Steven M. Haffner: Relationship of Metabolic Risk Factors and Development of Cardiovascular Disease and Diabetes. *Obesity* 14:121S-127S (2006) © 2006 The North American Association for the Study of Obesity.

Large adipocytes lead to the deposition of lipids in visceral and hepatic tissues promoting insulin resistance. Dietary calorie restriction, alone or with exercise, reverses this trend.

OSTEOPOROSIS

PREVALENCE: The use of dairy products to reduce osteoporosis and fractures has not panned out. Developed countries with the highest consumption of milk and cheese have high osteoporosis rates.

MEDICAL Rx: The ultimate goal is to reduce bone fractures, so in addition to adequate calcium the living bone tissue needs weight bearing exercises and enough vitamin D. There is constant bone resorption and bone rebuilding taking place in the skeleton and more resorption than rebuilding leads to osteoporosis. This is complicated by the fact that the metabolism of animal protein acidifies the blood leaching calcium from the bones as a buffer. Drugs used for osteoporosis attempt to decrease bone resorption, but unless we change the typical western diet high in dairy and meat to a non acidifying plant based diet, osteoporosis is here to stay.

NUTRITION APPROACH: Weight bearing exercises, enough Vitamin D, and adequate calcium intake, are top of the line approach for prevention and treatment of osteoporosis. Plant protein has proportionately less sulphur amino acids to acidify the blood than animal protein, so it does not leach calcium from the bones thereby naturally reducing bone resorption. Cow's milk is promoted as a calcium rich food, but the casein milk protein is the most relevant out of all the chemical carcinogens studied in the government's chemical carcinogen testing program, making it a less desirable source than calcium rich plants such as collards and cabbage. Because its protein is not paired with saturated fat, as it is in meat and dairy, a plant based diet is not associated with heart disease, so it wins again.

REFERENCES:

1. www.who.int/nutrition/topics/5 population nutritnt/en/indexx25html
The calcium recommendations of the Joint FAO/WHO Expert Consultation on Vitamin and Mineral Requirements in Human Nutrition highlights the following paradox: hip fracture rates are higher in developed countries where calcium intake is higher than in developing countries where calcium intake is lower. To date, the accumulated data indicate that the adverse effect of protein, in particular animal (but not vegetable) protein, might outweigh the positive effect of calcium intake on calcium balance. Mixed diets with emphasis on plants seem to have a favorable impact on bone in addition to many other benefits. The strength of evidence comes from fracture as outcome, rather than apparent bone mineral density as measured by dual-energy X-ray absorptiometry or other indirect methods. Excessive phosphorous in the meat diets of carnivores results in the kidneys' inability to reabsorb calcium. Low levels of calcium in the blood signal the parathyroid gland to solve the imbalance. Increased parathyroid hormone acts by removing calcium from the bones to replenish it in the blood stream. This provoked state of hyperparathyroidism causes decalcification of bone and pathological fractures. Moderate to vigorous physical activity is associated with hip fracture risk reduction of 38 to 45%.

2. Abelow BJ, Holford TR, Insogna KL: Cross-cultural association between dietary animal protein and hip fracture: a hypothesis. *Calcif Tissue Int.* 1992 Jan;50(1):14-8.
Abstract: Age-adjusted female hip fracture incidence has been noted to be higher in industrialized countries than in nonindustrialized countries. A possible explanation that has received little attention is that elevated metabolic acid production associated with a high animal protein diet might lead to chronic bone buffering and bone dissolution. In an attempt to examine this hypothesis, cross-cultural variations in animal protein consumption and hip fracture incidence were examined. When female fracture rates derived from 34 published studies in 16 countries were regressed against estimates of dietary animal protein, a strong, positive association was found. This association could not plausibly be explained by either dietary calcium or total caloric intake. Recent studies suggest that the animal protein-hip fracture association could have a biologically tenable basis. We conclude that further study of the metabolic acid-osteoporosis hypothesis is warranted.

3. Exercise interventions: defusing the world's osteoporosis time bomb. *Bulletin of the World Health Organization*: vol.81 no.11 Genebra Nov. 2003 Print ISSN 0042-9686.

4. David R Jacobs Jr and Maureen A Murtaugh: It's more than an apple a day: an appropriately processed, plant-centered dietary pattern may be good for your health. *Am J Clin Nutr* 2000;72:899–900.

5. Bone Health USDA Agricultural Research Service Grand Forks Human Nutrition Research Center Published in the *Journal of Clinical Nutrition* 2008. The World Health Organization emphasizes that "Physical activity is vital for maintaining healthy bones throughout life and is an important factor in preventing osteoporosis, reducing falls, and decreasing the risk of hip fractures. The alarming increase in prevalence of osteoporosis apparently expresses a pressing need for a more active lifestyle among people of all ages. The key benefits of regular physical activity have been well proven—the challenge to policy-makers and health professionals is to determine how to promote it among the general population. National and local policies should be developed and campaigns devised to improve public awareness of the need for active living, accompanied by well-conceived programmes to make physical activity easier and more rewarding. The best way we can help defuse the world's osteoporosis time bomb and prevent unnecessary suffering and mounting health care costs is by taking action now."

PAIN SYNDROMES/ MIGRAINE

PREVALENCE: Many variations of headaches are common worldwide and difficult to quantify.

MEDICAL Rx: Migraine, a recurrent throbbing headache often accompanied by nausea and vomiting, is best managed with prevention which includes a healthful lifestyle, regular sleep, timely eating, and less stress. Individualized treatment with medications may be necessary for some.

NUTRITIONAL APPROACH: The simple elimination of trigger foods can have a tremendous impact reducing or eliminating the headache in 20% to 50% of people. The top ten culprit foods in order of importance are: cheese, chocolate, eggs, citrus, meat, wheat, nuts, peanuts, tomatoes, and onions.

REFERENCES:
N Barnard: *Foods That Fight Pain*, New York; Harmony Books; 1998.

FOODBORNE ILLNESSES

The microorganisms that cause foodborne illnesses live inside the intestines of animals, which means that they transmit disease when your food or drink is contaminated with feces. Slaughterhouses (where cows, chickens, and turkeys go to be butchered) are all contaminated with feces and so is the meat. Eggs are contaminated not only by the hen's feces but as the egg forms inside her body. A meat and dairy centered diet poses a constant health risk and is unsustainable especially as the population grows.

PREVALENCE: The final report on the Global Burden of Foodborne Diseases will be released in 2015. Centers for Disease Control (CDC) estimates that each year roughly 48 million people (1 in 6 Americans) get sick, 128,000 are hospitalized, and 3,000 die of foodborne diseases. These cases include the obviously contaminated meat and eggs, but also plant crops contaminated by water runoff carrying the waste of animals downstream to the fruit or vegetable farm.

The following bacteria are most commonly implicated in foodborne diseases:

1. Campylobacter—up to 100% of poultry, including chickens, turkeys, and waterfowl have asymptomatic intestinal infections. The major reservoirs of the strain C. fetus are cattle and sheep.

2. Escherichia coli (commonly referred as E. coli) is found in the intestines of people and animals. The very toxic E. coli O157:H7 and other pathogenic E. coli mostly live in the intestines of cattle, but have also been found in the intestines of chickens, deer, sheep, and pigs. According to a study published in 2011, an estimated 93,094 illnesses are due to domestically acquired E. coli O157:H7 each year in the United States. Estimates of foodborne-acquired O157:H7 cases result in 2,138 hospitalizations and 20 deaths annually.

3. Salmonella commonly infects beef, poultry, milk, and eggs. In the United States, Salmonella infection causes more hospitalizations and deaths than any other germ found in food, resulting in direct medical costs of $365 million annually. Consuming improperly prepared or cooked eggs, poultry, or meat, raw milk or unpasteurized dairy products and juices poses a great risk.

Shigellosis rarely occurs in animals other than humans. The causative organism is frequently found in water polluted with human feces, and is transmitted via the fecal oral route.

MEDICAL Rx: Supportive treatment varies according to infection.

NUTRITIONAL APPROACH: Since plant foods do not have intestines they do not harbor the above bacteria. However they can get contaminated if they grow downstream from an animal farm or a meat processing facility. As long as people expect meat and cheese on their plate, everyone including plant eaters will be at risk of foodborne illnesses.

REFERENCE:
The Centers for Disease Control CDC and the World Health Organization WHO.

Enjoy the dawn of a new day in better health.

(NOTE: The next book you should read if you haven't already is *Whole: Rethinking the Science of Nutrition* by Professor T. Colin Campbell of *The China Study* with Howard Jacobson)

Part VI

Useful Information Plus Recipes

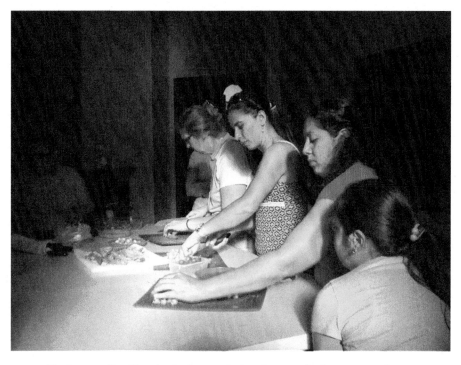

Cooking in Profile—bathed in sunlight, the sound of women cooking, teaching, nourishing the world.

30
Greens On a Budget

*G*reens *On A Budget* began in 2003 when I first met to cook with my patients. The name came out of a brief brainstorm with colleague Mary Wirshup. My assumption then was the same as today, that when delicious attractive whole plant foods are easy to use they push unhealthy items off the plate. The goal remains to use food as medicine by improving on food literacy. We started with basic recipes and altered them by adding different fruits to the oatmeal and different color vegetables to the salads. We prepare multigrain dishes, flavorful leafy greens, bean stews, baked roots, smooth and chunky soups. Participants get exposed to the enormous variety of nature's whole plant foods.

Twelve years later, armed with a dozen chopping boards and knives, we are still cooking. The group has settled on a permanent time which reduces confusion. We are mentioned in the free neighborhood paper and on the library website. We advertise in local restaurants, the Laundromat, and the community resource center, however most new participants come by word of mouth. Between four and twenty-four regularly attend, mostly women, children of all ages, and an occasional man. Children are often the reminders at home, which attests to the entertaining aspect of this learning activity. If we have left overs, we send an ambassador food sample home for those who stayed behind.

The gatherings are living sensory experiences where adults and children get exposed to the colors, aromas, and tastes of mother nature's harvest. Everyone enjoys the constant learning. For instance, that fruits get sweeter as they ripen. The opposite is true of many vegetables which are sweetest when they are young. We do not peel most fruits and vegetables, thereby encouraging many to start using whole plants. We make cooking with general rules less mysterious, for example grains and legumes all cook the same way in plenty of water. We strive to make the complicated simple. Everything in the produce aisle is edible, this means we don't need to know the name kohlrabi to take it home and taste it.

Personal and pleasant food memories are durable. You only find out how hard or heavy is a butternut squash when you pick one up. It's not easy to tell whether a mango is hard or too soft unless you touch it. The sweet smell of a pineapple gives away that it is ripe—this is important since pineapple will not continue to ripen when you bring it home. Bite a spicy daikon and you will immediately know it is not a white carrot. We use the kitchen as a laboratory and crack open a pomegranate, smell cinnamon, squirt lemon juice, add cilantro, watch rice swell, observe cooking time, and taste our dish in progress. The more experience one has with whole ingredients the more confidence in using them.

TV cooking shows may be entertaining and some offer valuable tips, but they naturally leave out touch, smell, and taste. Better roll up your sleeves and embark on our own food adventure. If you need coaching with an ingredient or a recipe and there is no one around, find a short tutorial on the internet. Gatherings where everyone participates in chopping and mixing can be transforming. Children like to imitate adults. Wash their hands up to their elbows and let them toss a salad with their bare hands, this method is likely to keep ingredients from flying out of the bowl. Let them measure ingredients and add them to the bowl or show them how to push buttons progressively on the blender. A plastic serrated knife initiates them in the safe use of an essential tool. Print educational materials that can spark lively conversations. You will find some at the end of this book, such as a sampling of whole plant foods, the amount of calcium in cabbage and collards, and the portion of foods which amount to 100 calories.

We use four main food groups: vegetables and leafy greens, grains, legumes, and fruits. We always include some brassica or cruciferous vegetables for their countless nutrients, vitamin C, fiber, and phytochemicals which help us with detoxification and cancer protection. In our workshops we practice cooking without flour, oil, and sugar—ingredients which are over emphasized in the American diet and which in excess negatively affect our health. For fat we crush olives, avocados, or cashews. To flavor a currie we add a splash of light coconut milk and we blend our own spices. We use no meat, chicken, milk, or cheese. We use little salt. To sweeten a dish we use whole dates, apples, and grapes. Since bread is used mostly as a filler we don't serve bread with the meal. Instead we fill our selves with delicious and nourishing food.

We make many dishes as one pot meals emphasizing the ease of cooking.

We mix garlic and other spices in the hot skillet, add greens, wilt and season, then serve over rice. We chop mounds of greens into soups and bean stews. We mix humus with shredded carrots; we use sliced daikon or kohlrabi instead of chips. We prepare salads with nutritious bok choy and napa cabbage instead of lettuce and we make burritos with napa leaves instead of tortillas.

Our recipes are templates for the imagination. After twelve years of Greens on a Budget workshops, we continue to discover old plants and new ways to enjoy them. Participants report how they build upon their experience at home. Organic neighborhood gardens often share their nourishing harvest with us. Most importantly, I always show up and don't cancel except for snow. Half of the health and wellness revolution consists of eating more plants; the other half consists on eliminating foods that hurt. However, the overarching whole consists on not giving up.

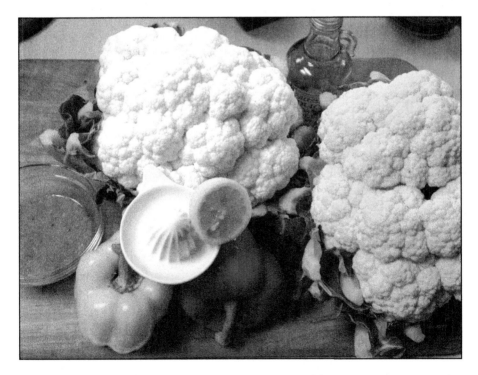

The Brassica family includes cauliflower and broccoli. Their inimitable shape and crunch when raw make them favorites among childrena and adults alike—this is prefect, since some of their healthful properties diminish with cooking.

31

My Human Body

*M*y Human Body: As I walk, talk, text, read, play, write, cook, wash, sit, sleep, daydream, breathe, my body quietly lives.

My body is an amazing organism in constant production, destruction, and repair.

It is responsible for the function of my skin, muscles, bones, and nerves; renews white and red blood cells, hormones and enzymes; repairs scrapes, wounds, and the intestinal lining; looks after my brain; gushes with tears, mucus, gastric juices, and saliva; is constantly growing hair and nails; makes cholesterol, bile, urine, stool, and myriad chemicals.

It tries to maintain a clutter free internal environment. After digesting oats, cookies, broccoli, or fries, it eliminates leftover waste; clears medicine from my system; destroys cells that have gone berserk or no longer work as a team. It sweeps the inside of arteries so my blood can flow freely; directs vitamins, antioxidants, and phytochemicals to vital tissues everywhere; turns inflammation on and then off on demand.

It is in constant communication with every part of itself: the feet with the hands, the thyroid with the pituitary, the pancreas with the mitochondria. It interacts with space, temperature, and surroundings. It can tell hostility from compassion and competition from group effort.

My body communicates with the whole organism and lets me know that I am tired, stressed, or satisfied, that I am awake, that I am hungry, that I need to pay bills, go to school, work, make dinner, or that I want to make love.

This organism counts on the nourishment I give it to sustain its day to day precious balance. It houses my self for life.

32

Composting

*Y*ou might ask why composting is included in this book. The reason is that maintaining an environment where resources are valued instead of wasted, channeling the refuse of worn out materials in support of more life and minding our immediate surroundings, is in essence very similar to mindfully caring for our bodies. Engaging in this physical practice can induce meditation, reduce stress, and help to remove obstacles from our way to greater health and wellness.

Composting is a simple household practice by which we can return organic matter to the soil.

As dead plants (and also animals) decompose they become soil again. This rich soil supports plant life which by extension supports all animal life. Organic humus from composting can be used for garden or house plants. Every time we compost organic matter instead of sending it to the landfill, we close the vital loop that restores circulation. Humans become involved in the process of composting by regularly discarding kitchen refuse in a designated place in the garden and harvesting rich humus in the end.

Organic waste that is picked up by the garbage truck pours nutrients and hard earned money into the landfill, where up to 60% is organic matter, such as grass clippings, yard refuse, and kitchen waste. These materials are capable of turning to soil, but in the landfill they cannot decompose. Surrounded by inert waste such as metal or plastic they stay intact in isolated pockets—tying up valuable space and resources for centuries.

What goes in your bin and what does not? Organic matter will decompose, whereas cement, glass, plastic, metal will not. Plant matter will render a sweet smelling compost, whereas fat and animal flesh will rot with an unpleasant odor, so keep meat and cheese out of the bin. The droppings of vegetable eating animals are valuable for your compost mix, whereas those of meat eaters, such as your dog or cat should be kept out.

Seeds are quite durable plant matter and should be kept out of the mix or they might sprout without your consent where you least expect them.

The kitchen to bin journey: Keep an open attractive 6 cup bowl by the sink for vegetable ends, fruit peels, coffee grinds, and tea bags. At least once a day take a short walk to the garden and empty it in the compost bin. Bins are sold online any time and at hardware stores during spring and summer. Look for a simple bin of durable construction and expect to pay about $150.

An ideal mix in the compost bin has more browns than greens in a proportion of about 2:1. This prevents excess moisture and allows for air to circulate throughout the material in the bin.

A bin filled with only dead dry brown leaves is very carbon rich. Although it will eventually decompose, it can remain a dry fluffy pile for a long time tying up your bin with little appreciable activity. If you have that many fallen leaves, pile them in a topless enclosure near your bin, scoops of them will help you balance a bin of mostly kitchen waste. Pile the rest in a corner of your yard and allow them to take their time.

A bin filled with kitchen waste is very nitrogen rich. It will also eventually decompose, but exclusively green kitchen waste could turn into a wet slime and tie up your bin for many months. Keep the balance by adding a layer of dry brown leaves every couple of weeks.

Helpful tips:

Large twigs and matted clumps of weeds will fill up your bin too quickly, they are best allowed to decompose in an open pile in some corner of your yard.

Minor imbalances inside the bin can greet you with fruit flies or a disagreeable smell when you open the lid to add new materials. To correct the situation immediately, just stir in some air and add a layer of dry brown leaves.

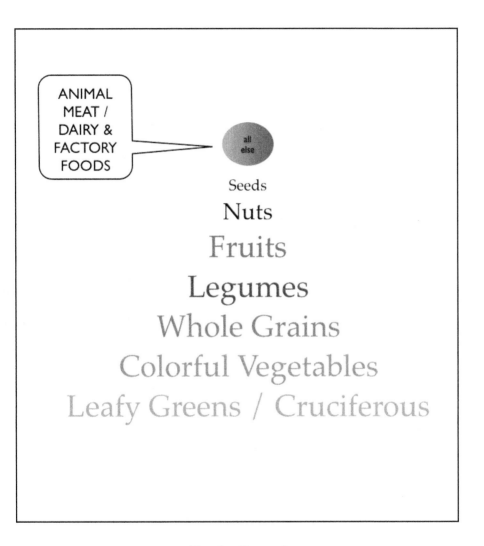

Timeless Pyramid

33
Calcium in Foods

The quantities detailed here are approximated to the nearest 0 or 5 milligrams (mg).

*W*e meet our calcium needs consuming a variety of nutrient rich plant foods. Leafy greens lose water and shrivel in the pot, which means you can fit even more calcium in a cup. On the other hand, grains and legumes absorb water in cooking which relative to its volume dilutes the calcium.

Calcium mg in	1 cup RAW	1 cup COOKED
VEGETABLES		
Arugula	30	100
Bok Choy / Napa Cabbage	45-75	165
Broccoli / Brussels Sprouts	35-40	55-70
Carrots / Potatoes / Cauliflower		20-35
Chinese Cabbage (Napa)	60	160
Collards / Mustard Greens	50-60	100-150
Kale, Turnip & Beet Greens, Okra	80-95	165-175
Sweet Potato/ Squash		70-80

SEA VEGETABLES
Arame, Hijiki, Wakame   1 cup dry, 400 mg

GRAINS
Quinoa   1 cup cooked, 100 mg

LEGUMES COOKED, 1 cup
Lima / Adzuki: 50-65
Chickpeas / Pinto Beans / Kidney: 80-90
Black (Turtle) Beans, Great Northern: 100-120
Navy / Vegetarian Baked Beans: 130
Soybeans: 175

NUTS AND SEEDS RAW, 1 oz
Sunflower / Walnuts: 20-25
Pistachio / Sesame: 40
Almonds : 75

FRUITS RAW
1 banana: 5
1 pear / 1 medium fig: 20-30
1 orange: 50
1 papaya: 70

TOFU, 4 oz or 1/5 of a block
Soft to Extra Firm: 195-270
Tempeh 4 oz: 225

NON-DAIRY MILKS (Fortified), 1 cup
Rice Dream Enriched: 300
Soy Dream Enriched: 300
Edensoy Extra: 200

OTHER BEVERAGES (Fortified), 1 cup
Orange Juice: 300

DAIRY, 1 cup
Whole Cow's Milk / Yogurt: 275
Cheddar cheese 1 oz: 100
Human Milk for comparison: 80

34

*Grains **already cooked.***

AMARANTH

1/4 CUP: 200 calories
36 grams of carbohydrate = 144 calories
7 grams of protein = 28 calories
3.2 g of fat = 28 calories

1/2 CUP: 400 calories
70 g of carbohydrate = 280 calories
14 g of protein = 56 calories
7 g of fat = 63 calories

CORN

1/2 CUP: 90 calories
17 g of carbohydrate = 69 calories
2.5 g of protein = 10 calories
1 g of fat = 9 calories

1 CUP: 177 calories
35 g of carbohydrate = 139 calories
5 g of protein = 20 calories
2 g of fat = 18 calories

MILLET

1/2 CUP: 200 calories
39 g of carbohydrate = 154 calories
6 g of protein = 24 calories
2.4 g of fat = 22 calories

1CUP: 400 cal
78 g of carbohydrate = 308 calories
12 g of protein = 48 calories
5 g of fat = 45 calories

OATS

1/2 CUP: 75 calories
13 g of carbohydrate = 54 calories
3 g of protein = 12 calories
1 g of fat = 9 calories

1 CUP: 150 calories
26 g of carbohydrate = 108 calories
6 g of protein = 24 calories
2.3 g of fat = 18 calories

QUINOA

1/2 CUP: 150 cal
26 g carbohydrate = 103 calories
6 g protein = 24 calories
2.5 g fat = 23 calories

1 CUP: 300 cal
52 g carbohydrate = 206 calories
12 g protein= 48 calories
5 g fat = 45 calories

RICE

1/2 CUP: 100 cal
20 g carbohydrate = 80 calories
2-3 g protein = 12 calories
1 g fat = 9 calories

1 CUP: 200 cal
40 g carbohydrate = 162 calories
4-5 g protein= 20 calories
1-2 g fat = 18 calories

WHEAT

1/2 CUP: 75 calories
16 g carbohydrate = 63 calories
3 g protein = 12 calories
0 g fat

1 CUP: 150 calories
32 g carbohydrate = 128 calories
6 g protein = 24 calories
<1/2 g fat = 0

Most grains are the compact seeds of grasses. They store enough calories to eventually germinate and push above ground where the seedling can start making its own carbohydrate, proteins, and fat.

Most quinoa sold commercially in North America is processed or bred to remove a bitter resinous saponin coating that would have required vigorous rinsing before cooking. In its natural form, this chemical makes the plant unpopular with birds and insects.

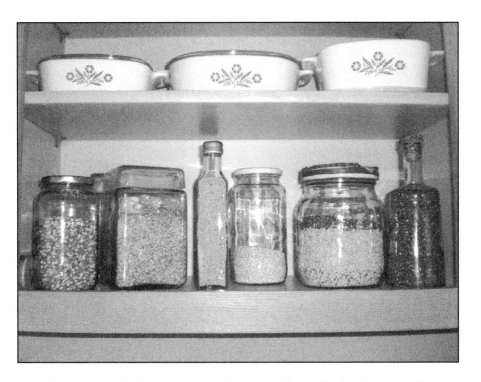

Whole grains retain their nutritious oily germ and bran which when exposed to air get oxidized and turn rancid. Keep them in transparent jars inside the cupboards. Refill jars only when empty to ensure freshness. Do not mix different age seeds. From left to right: corn, brown rice, amaranth, barley, steel cut oats, and red quinoa. (The grains which contain gluten are—barley, rye, oats processed with other grains, and all varieties of wheat such as kamut, spelt, and farro.)

35

Portions Equal to 100 Calories

To be food literate means to be competent and knowledgeable about what we eat. The following list of foods is arranged alphabetically in amounts equal to 100 calories. These do not represent normal portions, but only a comparison of amounts and calories. In other words, it is practical to know that a tablespoon of oil has more calories than 5 cups of salad greens. Likewise it is helpful to know that one ounce of cheese has the same amount of calories as 3 cups of squash. Understanding food at this level helps one better balance calorie intake.

apple or grapefruit, 1 medium
avocado, 1/4 fruit
banana, 1 medium
beans cooked, 1/2 to 1 cup
blueberries, 1 1/4 cup
bread or bagel, 1 slice or 3 inches in diameter
broccoli, 2 cups
Brussels sprouts, 2 cups
cabbage, 5 cups
carrots, 1 1/2 cups
cauliflower, 3 cups
chocolate, 3/4 ounce semi sweet
cheese, 1 ounce
chestnuts, 5 nuts
collards, 2 cups
corn, 1 cup
cranberries fresh unsweetened, 2 cups
egg, 1 1/2 egg
flour (white or whole), 1/4 cup
garlic, 25 cloves
lemon juice, 1 cup
meat (chicken, beef, pork, fish), 1 ounce (1.5 x 2 inches)

melon, 2 cups

milk almond, 2 cups unsweetened

milk 1 % cow, 1 cup

mushrooms, 5 cups

nuts: almonds, cashews, pistachios, walnuts, peanuts, 3/4 ounce (10-15
  pieces)

oats, 3/4 cup

okra, 1 cup

olives black, 8 super colossal

olive oil, 2 1/2 teaspoons

orange, 2 medium

orange juice, 1 cup

pasta, 1/2 cup

pear and plums, 1 medium or 2 fruits

rice, 1/2 cup

salad greens, 5 cups

salmon, 1 1/2 ounces

scallions, 3 cups chopped

sesame seeds, 6 teaspoons = 2 tablespoons

soy beans, 1/2 cup

squash and zucchini, 3 cups

36

Common Vegan Sources of Fat

$\mathcal{W}$e need less than 20% of our calories from fat each day. By keeping a lose mental count of fat intake we can easily stay within these healthful limits. If a cookie is 100 calories and has 2 grams of fat then 18% of its calories come from fat. If a Danish is 240 calories and has 10 grams of fat then 37% of its calories are from fat. A plant based vegan does not need to worry, but if your diet consists mainly of processed food, watch out.

Amount	Total Calories:	Fat Calories:	% Fat:
Any oil, 1 Tablespoon	120 calories	120	100%
1 cup = 16 TBS	1920 calories	1920	100%

Olive oil confers little or no benefit unless we have significantly reduced fat in the diet to around 15%.

Edamame 4 Oz: 1/2 cup:	160 calories	65	41%
Tofu 2.5 Oz: 1/5 block:	80 calories	35	43%
Tempeh 4 Oz: 1/2 block:	240 calories	100	42%
Nuts / Seeds 1/4 C; 1 oz:	165 calories	110	66%
Avocado 1/2 Fruit:	150 calories	135	90%
Olives 6:	75 calories	56	75%
Vegenaise™ 1 tbs:	90 calories	80	88%
Humus Oil Free 2 tbs:	30 calories	25	83%
Ice Cream			50%
Cheese 1 oz:	90 calories	63	70%
Vegan Choc Chips 1 tbs:	70 calories	36	51%
Coconut Milk 1/2 cup:	70 calories	60	85%
V Choc Cake 1 slice:	244 calories	86	35%
Bakery Items	Variable		

37
Legumes: Beans, Peas, And Lentils

Legumes or beans are seeds that grow in pods. Like most plants they are low in calories, rich in carotenes, lutein, vitamin C, folate, B vitamins, carbohydrates, and fiber.

Fresh green beans are rich in Beta carotene, lutein, zeaxanthine, and vitamin C. Mature dry beans are rich in protein, complex carbohydrates, B vitamins, like folate and thiamin, minerals like potassium, magnesium, selenium, iron, and fiber. Aim to eat a cup of legumes each day.

HOW TO BUY:

Fresh beans are seasonal, buy canned or frozen any time.
Look for sugar snap peas that are plump and they will be sweet and tender.
Buy dry beans from places with a brisk turnover. Inspect the bags and refuse those with broken or powdery contents.

HOW TO STORE:

Fresh beans: refrigerate immediately because within six hours at room temperature half of the delicious sugars will turn to starch.
Dry beans: store sealed in a cool dry place.
Cooked beans: keep in refrigerator for a week or longer in the freezer.

HOW TO COOK:

Lentils do not need soaking and will cook in 30 to 45 minutes.
Inspect dry beans for pebbles by spreading them on a towel.
Soak them in water for at least 6 hours (overnight) before cooking.
Rinse again to remove gas forming oligosacharides then cook in fresh water until tender.
After they are soft, season to taste.
Fresh legumes: steam or eat raw.

SERVING SUGGESTIONS:

Fold bean sprouts into salads, dips, and spreads.

Add frozen or fresh peas to a salad or to a cooked casserole.

Steam fresh beans and puree with a few drops of olive oil, garlic, salt, and fresh herbs.

Add home cooked or canned legumes to soups, stews, or casseroles.

Combine cooked beans with garlic, onions, tomatoes, chopped kale, and sweet potato, then season well and serve on top of rice.

Mash cooked beans into a potato salad.

Cook beans in a spiced broth, mash, and use as spread or dip.

Stir fry cooked beans with colorful vegetables and experiment with a variety of seasonings, such as coconut, cumin, rosemary, oregano, cilantro, ginger, for different ethnic flavors.

Add fresh or cooked beans to salad greens.

Add beans to pasta sauce.

Combine seasoned mashed beans with cooked rice for vegetarian patties.

Toss steamed shell beans with lemon and onion.

Toss warm cooked lentils in a vinaigrette.

TROUBLESHOOTING:

Tough skin: cook next time in plain water, do not add acid seasoning like tomato, vinegar, or lemon juice, until after the beans are tender.

Remove leathery fava skin before cooking for a delicious tender bean.

Gas: soak for at least 6 hours and rinse then cook until tender and rinse again to remove oligosacharides that ferment in our gut causing gas.

38
A More Nourishing Community Food Pantry

Build a Community Food Pantry as you would your own
with selections such as these.

1. Minimally processed canned foods:
One ingredient on the label, canned in water, or in their own juice.Large
cans of cooked beans, large cans of diced or stewed tomatoes, plain
tomato sauce, canned corn or pumpkin, jars of peanut butter (no oil or
sugar added).
2. Milk drinks:
Cartons of unsweetened soy, almond, and rice milks, low in fat and calcium
rich.
3. Bagged dry goods:
Brown or white rice; and dry beans like red, pink, black, chickpeas, navy,
lentils, and others.
Corn grits, rolled or steel cut oats, buckwheat or groats, barley, quinoa.
Plain wheat pasta and gluten free pasta from rice, corn, or quinoa.
4. Nuts and seeds:
Raw or dry roasted nuts, such as almonds, walnuts, cashews, pistachios.
Inspect the label and avoid nuts roasted in oils with added salt and
sugars which, makes them a very high calorie item.
5. Condiments:
Buy in jars, in plastic or tin containers, or in bulk. Condiments are essential
in preparing savory meals with any produce fresh or frozen.
Garlic paste, olives, capers, lemon juice, roasted red peppers, black pepper,
and ground oregano, parsley, dill, mustard, ginger, cumin...
6. Kitchen essentials:
Consider providing tools of the trade. Even the best intentioned cannot
cook without a chopping board, a sharp vegetable knife, a measuring
cup, some bowls, a blender, basic stainless steel pots, pans, spoons, and a
ladle.

Minimize:

Factory processed foods come conveniently bagged or boxed and might
be essential for people without access to a kitchen, but read the labels
for fillers like flour, sugar, corn syrup, oils, artificial flavors, colors, and
preservatives. These items—breads, boxed cereals, and pastries; instant
soups and potatoes; canned cheese pasta, sweet pork and beans, syrup
canned fruit, and sweet drinks or juices—supply calories without many
nutrients and are associated with heartburn, promote high sugar, high
cholesterol, obesity, and heart disease. Choose mindfully.

39
Household Suggestions

Frequent comments regarding healthful eating include: It takes too much time! My children won't try anything new. I don't know where to begin. Junk food is everywhere! I don't seem able to stick with healthful changes. My friends show no interest. These thoughts block the most important change of all: our own individual attitude. Imagine yourself diligently removing these mental roadblocks. Without this step, we stay stuck.

Do not compare yourself to anyone else. Wherever you are, there is where you begin! Choose an activity that seems easy for you and build on success. Practice it. Start with one of these:

— I will start making rolled oats instead of instant oats.

__One morning this week I will make steel cut oats.

__One night I will take 90 seconds to measure 1/2 cup steel cut oats for each one in the house and soak them overnight in a pan with water. In the morning, I will set the timer and cook the oats for 10 minutes!

__The first person down for breakfast will cut an apple in small cubes, sprinkle it with cinnamon, and add it to the oatmeal. The aroma might entice the no-breakfast-for-me person.

Include household members as you embark in changes that affect them. Build upon whole foods already used. For example:

__Draw a plate on a large piece of cardboard (20 inches across). Divide it up in quadrants using the Colorful Plate and The Sustainable Plate Tables as guides. Cut out and paste pictures of what you or your family eat from each group. Observe the proportion of your choices. Keep this poster visible and expand your choices of whole grains, fruits, green leafy vegetables, roots, and other colorful vegetables, legumes, seeds and nuts.

__On your next trip to the grocery store, ask the child or yourself to select a new leafy green vegetable from the produce stand. When back at home try it raw, steamed, in a stew, stir fried, and record the family's response. If it wins approval, add it to the household plate.

Experiment with a new spice this month. Spices loose their fragrance if stored too long, so buy a small jar and use it! Swap small amounts purchased in bulk with a friend.
__For dessert or a snack, core apples and stud them with spice cloves, place a cinnamon stick in the center. Cook in a covered pan with an inch of water until the desired consistency. Sweet delight!

As we invest creative energy in food preparation, we assume responsibility for our own health care.

SAMPLING OF WHOLE FOODS
Adapted from: www.greensonabudget.org

Make unrefined foods 90% of your diet. Enjoy both raw and cooked with minimal processing. Stimulate your taste buds. These leafy greens and colorful vegetables have phytochemicals that protect our health. Free of fat, they are filled with water, vitamins, minerals, and anti-oxidants. Their cellulose fiber body acts like a sponge in our intestines retaining moisture and dragging away waste. The variety in colors suggests plants abundant nutrition. Dare to try something new and different.

Fruits are a delicious way to include even more variety of flavor and nutrition. Combine them with other plants, sprinkle with a fistful of nuts or ground flax seeds and taste your new dish.

Nuts and seeds are nutrient rich. Remember that within them are all the concentrated ingredients for the sprout to push its way through the ground until it reaches sunlight and can make its own food. Use them sparingly.

Eat an unlimited amount of leafy greens. 1 pound is roughly 100 calories:
kale, collards, bok choy, cabbage, Napa Brussels sprouts, watercress,

turnip greens, broccoli raab, Swiss chard. lettuces (Romaine or equivalent), beet greens, dandelion greens, escarole, spinach.

Eat large amounts of colorful vegetables each day:
asparagus, artichokes, snow peas, string beans, sprouts, zucchini, chayote, cucumbers, okra, broccoli, cauliflower, eggplants, red peppers, tomatoes, nopales (cactus pads), water chestnuts.

Eat a cup of heavy solid vegetables a day:
daikon radish, turnips, kohlrabi, rutabaga, carrots, beets, potatoes, sweet potatoes, pumpkins, butternut, acorn squash, taro root, malanga.

Eat a cup of cooked legumes or beans a day:
chickpeas, navy beans, moth beans, black eyed peas, black beans, pinto beans, lentils, mung beans, red kidney beans, pigeon peas, cannellini, peanuts and soybeans (both similar in fat to nuts).

Eat a cup of cooked whole grains a day:
corn, rice (many varieties brown and white), amaranth, millet, buckwheat, wild rice, oats - whole grain / flattened flakes, quinoa; wheat, rye, barley: only grains with gluten.

Eat a total of 4 cups of various fruits a day:
apples, apricots, bananas, raspberries, strawberries, blueberries, dates, figs, cranberries, grapes, kiwis, mangoes, persimmons, papayas, pineapples, melons, pears, nectarines, peaches, plums, oranges, tangerines.

Eat no more than 20 raw nuts or one tablespoon of seeds a day. One ounce is roughly 100 calories.
chestnuts (more similar to legumes), almonds, cashews, walnuts, coconut, pine nuts (pignolis), pecans, pistachios, macadamias, pumpkin seeds, sesame seeds, sunflower seeds, flax seeds (ground).

40

Recipes

*B*rassica vegetables, also known as Cruciferous vegetables for their cross-shaped flowers are a large group of vegetables which includes Arugula, Broccoli, Cauliflower, Brussels Sprouts, Cabbage, Watercress, Bok Choy, Turnip Greens, Mustard Greens, Collard Greens, Rutabaga, Napa or Chinese Cabbage, Radishes such as Daikon, Turnips, Kohlrabi, and Kale. Chemical substances found in these vegetables stimulate detoxification by the liver and assist in the break down of potential carcinogens. These properties help to maintain the integrity of the tumor protective gene p53, therefore protect normal cells, help delay the onset of some cancers, and reduce the size and growth of tumors. The chemicals in Brassica vegetables help keep our blood clean and reduce the levels of homocysteine which is an inflammatory marker associated with a higher risk of cardiovascular disease.

The less cooked, the more you benefit from the active phytochemicals, since they break down when exposed to prolonged heat. For example: 34% of the sulforaphanes available in raw broccoli are reduced to 4% when fully cooked. Having said this, do not get stuck on this notion, some is more than nothing. Prepare them in your favorite way and consume generous amounts.

Suggestions: Bake cabbage leaves stuffed with beans, rice, mushrooms, and other colorful vegetables; sauté them in garlic with a drizzle of olive oil; grind broccoli or cauliflower and add to mashed potatoes or sweet potatoes; stir fry leafy greens with other vegetables, bake them or roast them and enjoy their sweetness by themselves or with added flavorful herbs and spices.

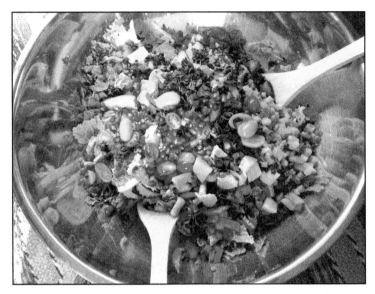

A rainbow salad in its infinite permutations is limited only by the imagination.

RAINBOW SALAD

Prepare enough for 3 to 4 days. As the greens begin to wilt, stir fry it in the skillet with slices of squash, sweet potato, eggplant, or artichokes; or add it to the pot of beans you prepared that week! Do not let your salad go to waste.

Practice making your own dressing using 2 or 3 of these ingredients in any combination: lemon juice, vinegar, water, olive oil, salt, pepper, ketchup, Vegenaise (a soy based mayo), ginger, or chipotle—don't add it until ready to eat. Use only enough dressing to coat your salad and enhance its flavor never drown it. Every bite will be a different experience. The flavors of ingredients chopped small leave each piece and help savor the whole.

One whole napa (Chinese) cabbage

Half a bunch cilantro (5 sprigs)

Cucumbers: 1 or 2

Red pepper: one large

Green onions: 5 or 6

Mushrooms: two cups

Garlic: a few minced cloves

A cup or two of cooked beans: sample the enormous variety, not just garbanzos

Add an orange and other diced fruit: pear, mango, pomegranate seeds, etc.

Add carrots, cauliflower, broccoli, slices of avocado

Add a fistful of almonds, walnuts, or a sprinkle of sesame seeds.

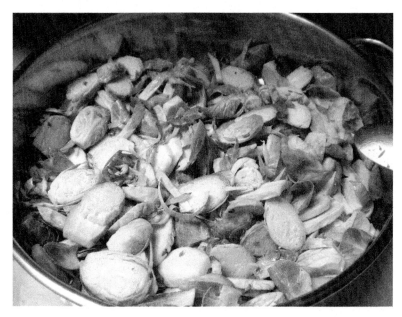

Brussels sprouts with fennel seeds—if you avoid these little cabbages from the Brassica family because of past unappetizing experiences, this is the dish to try.

BRUSSELS SPROUTS AND FENNEL SEEDS

2 tablespoons fennel seeds
1 tablespoon oil
1 pound Brussels sprouts cut in 0.25 inch
   slices
Salt and pepper
Balsamic or rice vinegar
Water

Gently warm the oil and fennel seeds in a large skillet for about 5 minutes until fragrant.
Turn up the heat to medium then add the sprouts all at once and sprinkle with salt and pepper.
Toss with the seeds, add a couple of tablespoons of water, and immediately cover to trap the water vapor.
Steam the sprouts covered medium high for about 5 minutes. They should be cooked while retaining a bright green color.
Check for tenderness before removing from the heat.
Arrest the cooking by transferring them to a cold plate.
Add a couple of teaspoons of vinegar and toss. (Balsamic vinegar will slightly darken the dish, sherry or rice vinegar will not.)
Hot or cold these little cabbages are delicious.

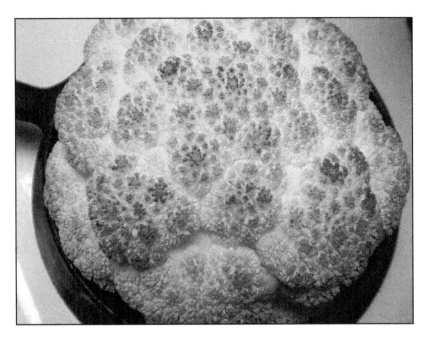

A baked cauliflower trades the availability of some of its nutrients with the
mouthwatering sensation of crispy on the outside and tender moist on the inside.
Position the whole cauliflower in a dry ovenproof pan with no water, no oil,
no seasonings, and bake uncovered at 400° for one hour. Break off pieces
at the table as you woud a loaf of bread.

BAKED MARINATED CAULIFLOWER OR BROCCOLI

1 head of cauliflower and / or broccoli
separated into florets

1 red and 1 yellow bell peppers cut in quarter
inch strips

Marinade, whisk it separately, and drizzle
over the vegetables:

The juice of 2 large lemons plus 1 Tbs olive
oil

1 tsp sherry vinegar (optional)

1 tsp cumin

1 tsp coriander

Salt and Pepper

Spread the dry vegetables single layer
in an ovenproof pan (e.g. Pyrex©).
Don't add any other liquid except the
marinade. Bake at 400° for one hour
until they look roasted crisp not burnt.
Remove from the oven, while still hot
add a layer of chopped fresh cilantro,
and inhale! Eat it hot, as a cold side
dish, take it to work or school.

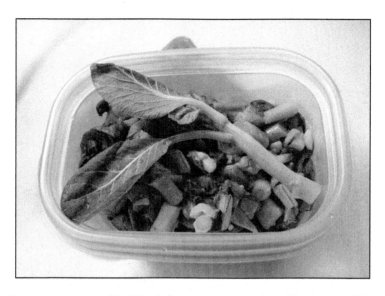

Lunch size containers of healthy delicious greens, such as these steamed broccoli tips, can improve your work eating experience.

LEAFY GREEN STIR FRY

Any leafy green lends itself to this quick preparation. Use kale, collards, Swiss chard, spinach, cabbages like napa or bok choy, beet greens, Asian mustard greens (not as sharp as regular mustard greens), or broccoli tips.

Method: To a medium warm skillet add 4-5 minced garlic cloves. In a teaspoon of water or olive oil, heat for a few minutes until the garlic is fragrant. Add a large bunch of chopped leafy greens. Sprinkle them with salt and pepper to enhance the flavor. Stir and toss for 5 to 10 minutes. Do not over cook to conserve nutrients and maintain their beautiful color. Serve over cooked rice, on top of a corn tortilla, wrapped in a cabbage or collard leaf, or all by itself.

Variations: Instead of oil try a few mashed olives; use light coconut milk with cumin or curry powder for a Thai flavor, experiment with ginger and other spices that smell good to you. If you are in the mood, separate the dish into several bowls and use a pinch of various herbs to see how you like them and take notes. Add these recipes to the cook book you already own.

Combinations: Cook cubed vegetables in the skillet before adding the greens; for example mushrooms, carrots, eggplant, squash, red pepper. Add more tender ingredients such as green peas, edamame (young soy beans), tomato, and cilantro, at the end.

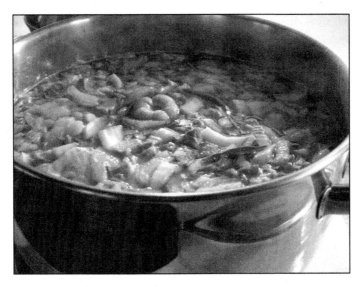

A stew of Navy beans with Napa cabbage, various root vegetables, and no oil.
Floating on top are a hot pepper, a bay leaf, and a slice of tomatillo
(citrus flavored tomato fruit)

BEANS STEW WITH KALE AND RICE

Many people find cooking dry beans intimidating. It could not be simpler.
Soak dry beans in plain water overnight. Keep refrigerated. If the soaked beans
have to wait more than a day for you to set the timer, change the water daily
to keep it fresh. Whenever you are ready; cook the soaked beans for one to two
hours in a pot of plain water. If you add condiments at this stage, the skins may
stay tough. Use the same method for any of your favorite beans. Cooking time
depends on the size of the beans (less than an hour for lentils and over two
hours for chickpeas). As dry beans rehydrate they swell and more than double in
size, so choose a pot that is large enough.

　　When you can easily squish them between your fingers, they are done!
Add running fresh water to overflow the pot and therefore rinse the beans of the
foamy starches that could ferment in your gut and give you gas. With enough
water to generously cover the beans, add the rest of the ingredients. You need a
large pot!

A large bunch of greens (one to two pounds) chopped into medium chunks: kale, collards,

Napa cabbage, bok choy, spinach, or callaloo (amaranth leaves typical in Caribbean dishes).
A small chopped bunch of herbs: cilantro, basil, parsley, or dill.
Mince an onion and several (four or five) garlic cloves. Try vegetable bullion or minced ginger.
Cube a variety of vegetables to suit your taste: sweet potato, pumpkin, carrots, red pepper, mushrooms, fresh or canned tomatoes, even half an apple or pear.

Simmer until vegetables are a little soft and the flavors have mingled. Season with salt, pepper, cumin, vinegar, tamarind, and/or molasses until satisfied. Experiment with different flavors and record your preferences.

Mash half cup of the beans for a thicker sauce. In my homeland Puerto Rico this versatile dish prepared with any number of legumes is served on top of rice.

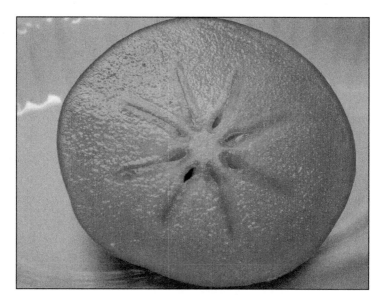

Look for the tomato shaped Fuyu persimmon—it is very sweet and non astringent.
A very nice treat.

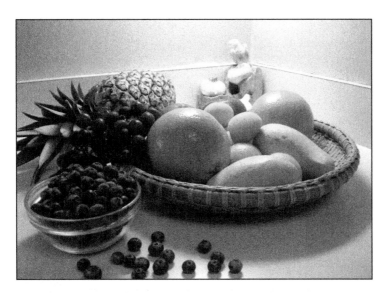

The sight and smell of ripening fruit changes with each season.
Perishable as they are, watch them closely to enjoy their peak. Do not let them go to
waste, these are nature's proud offspring. Keep a diced mix in a large bowl inside
the refrigerator for a delectable snack anytime.

FRUIT MEDLEY

This is a salad made of bite size pieces of fruits. Cut apples, pears, mangos,
pineapples, and melons, in half inch cubes to match the size of grapes cut in half.
Add pomegranate seeds and slices of star fruit. The salad will keep for a few days
if you start off with the sturdier fruits and add the berries, the bananas, or the
kiwis upon serving. A fruit medley invites anyone to a sweet refreshing serving
instead of to sugary popsicles or ice cream. Create your own combination based
of seasonal fruits.

FROZEN FRUIT TREASURES

During the summer we have access to much fruit. Bring home a bucket full.
Rinse lightly and air dry. Slice into blender friendly chunks. Arrange in single
layer on a cookie sheet and freeze overnight. Pop the frozen chunks into zip
lock bags (once frozen they will not stick to each other) and keep in the freezer.
Enjoy later as frozen pops or use them to make fruit smoothies, pancake
dressing, or puddings and jams.

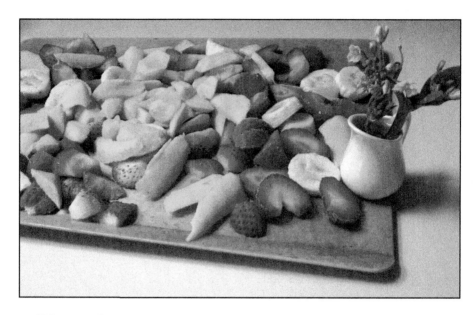

When ripe fruit is in abundant supply, wash, cube, and freeze, for a few hours then pop them in zip locked bags to later use in smoothies. A single layer as they freeze keeps the pieces from sticking together in a lump.

SMOOTHIES

Blend your favorite mix of frozen fruit with unsweetened calcium rich almond milk. Add a few leaves of raw kale, you won't even notice them and they will add even more nutrients to your treat.

CHIA SEED PUDDING, JAM, AND DRESSING

This omega rich seed has a dehydrated outer capsule which absorbs liquid like a sponge thickening any medium. Combine whole chia seeds with a little soy milk and frozen berries then let them sit for at least an hour in the refrigerator and enjoy a creamy pudding. Mix chia seeds with raw crushed fruit and they make a good jam or fruit salad dressing.

OATS: The simple difference between rolled oats and steel cut oats is in how they were processed. Steel cut oats are the raw whole grain cut into pieces. Rolled oats are steamed whole grains which have been flattened and then toasted dry. By weight they both have the same nutritional value. Steel cut oats take up less space than big fluffy rolled oat flakes and can absorb more water than rolled oats, which explains why you need 0.25 cup of steel cut oats compared to 0.5 cup of rolled oats to get a cup of cooked porridge. Because steel cut oats are more dense, a scanty 0.25 cup weighs the same as 0.5 cup of fluffy rolled oats. Okay, now choose the oats you prefer. Cook them in water with ground cinnamon then add fresh or frozen fruits and top with ground flax seeds. Eat them often for breakfast. Avoid the packets of instant flavored oatmeal—they have added sugars and are more expensive.

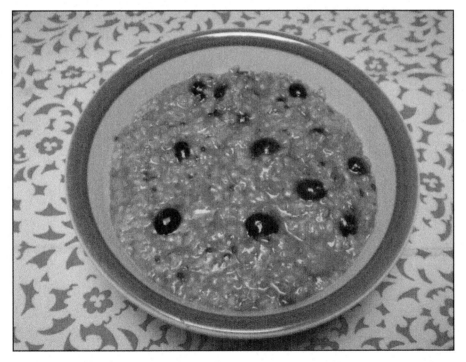

Steel cut oats cooked with quinoa for twenty minutes then sweetened with a handful of blueberries, but any fruit of your liking will do. A nutritious breakfast that will keep you satisfied all morning.

OATS AND QUINOA WITH FRUIT

Steel cut oats are raw whole grains that have been chopped into two or three pieces using a steel blade. They have not been steamed or rolled (flattened). Steel cut oats don't have more nutrition, but they add a chewy consistency to your breakfast. Keep a combination of dry oats and quinoa in a jar ready to scoop out. (One cup oats to one tablespoon quinoa) See Grains.

A quarter cup raw will turn into 3/4 cup when cooked and will keep you satisfied until lunch time.

Add: 1 cup of water and a drizzle of rice milk, almond milk, or soy milk for taste and calcium.

Half teaspoon of ground cinnamon

Half teaspoon of sugar is optional

Combine all the ingredients in a saucepan and cook uncovered at medium heat for 20 minutes.

Like all other grains oats cook until tender as they absorb water, so don't allow them to dry until fully done.

Turn off the heat and immediately add 1/2 cup of diced frozen or seasonal fresh fruit and berries. They contribute vitamins, fiber, sweetness, and color to your breakfast. Let sit for a minute until the fruit is warm. Avoid dried fruit. They are often sweetened with added sugars and since they are dehydrated we tend to underestimate the amount we use.

Sprinkle a teaspoon or two of ground flax seeds for their omega 3 fatty acids.

Practice this dish until it's just right for you and savor.

COOKIES

Mix 8 medium Medjool dates pitted and diced and 1/2 cup chopped pecans in the food processor.

Add 1/4 cup strawberries, 1/2 diced apple, 2 inches of banana and blend well.

Using the pulsing button fold 1 cup or more of rolled oats (not instant) until they are mixed uniformly in the dough.

Add dashes of allspice and cumin plus a pinch of cayenne pepper (do not overdo it).

Make 1.5 inch discs and place close to each other on a cookie sheet. Cook at 400° for almost 20 minutes.

Let cool. You may freeze them in a closed container for weeks. Makes about 4 dozen cookies.

DATE BALLS

Start with Medjool dates, pecans, and walnuts as above.

Process until a coarse crumble. Do not continue to a paste! The nuts are very oily and you will end with an utter mess.

Fold a couple of teaspoons of unsweetened cocoa powder and the rind of a large orange.

Make small 1 inch balls and roll them on ground coconut shavings, this keeps them from sticking with each other.

Arrange in a pyramid on a small platter. Average serving is two balls per person.

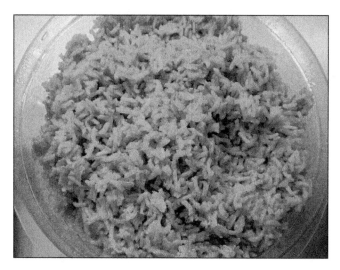

Brown rice can be coaxed out of its dull looks with colorful condiments, such as turmeric, saffron, paprika, or a few drops of anato (achiote seeds) dyed oil.

SAVORY GRAINS

Cook the grains separately and keep them in the refrigerator for use during the week.

Rice: try various varieties of brown rice but could use any kind.

Quinoa: toast lightly on a dry pan then cook about twenty minutes.

Wheat berries: this large hard grain takes about an hour to cook.

Spelt: combined with other wheats it is called farro—lower in gluten, but not gluten free. Cooks in 45 minutes.

Corn: fresh or canned no salt or sugars added. Does not need cooking.

Combine in a large bowl and add the following savory ingredients for a colorful nutritious dish.

Tomato diced

Juice of one large lemon

Cilantro chopped: up to 1 1/2 cups

Season with salt and pepper to taste.

Enjoy the colors, textures, and flavors. The lemon juice will help release the cilantro aroma. Pack a cup for work or school as part lunch. Watch the reaction of others as you open your aroma filled container...share the recipe. Use various combinations as a side to stir fries; add to stews or soups.

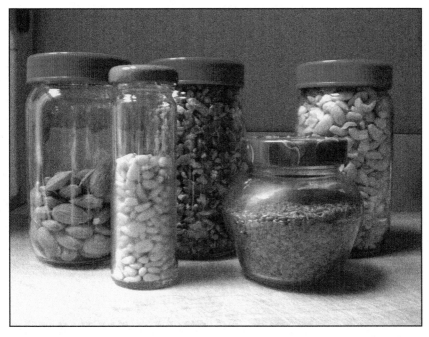

Nuts like grains, are also seeds. Keep small amounts to ensure freshness. From right to left: cashews, flax seeds, pecans, pine nuts, and almonds.

LENTIL SALAD

1 pound French lentils
1 unsalted vegetable bullion cube

Cook the lentils in ample vegetable broth until tender but still firm, for about 30 minutes
Drain the lentils and keep the broth for a soup or some other dish.
Add to the cooked lentils:

2-3 carrots diced the size of the lentils
2 celery stalks diced the size of lentils
1 red pepper diced as above
2-3 tablespoons chopped fresh dill
2-3 tablespoons chopped fresh tarragon
2-3 tablespoons chopped fresh parsley

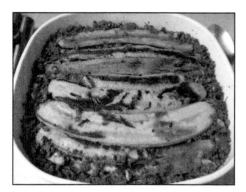 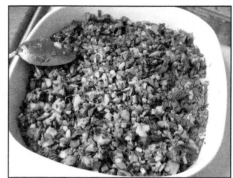

A "pastelón" of ripe plantains, soy meat stuffing, and mounds of chopped greens resembles a lasagna. Simply put it consists of layers in a pan. Except for the greens tossed in you favorite seasonings, everything is already cooked. Forty minutes to an hour in the oven will bring the flavors together.

FILLING FOR TYPICAL DISHES SUCH AS PASTELES, PIONONOS, AND TAMALES

Cook in a large pot adjusting the ingredients to the size of your party:

Garlic cloves minced
Onion or scallions chopped
Red pepper diced
Crushed tomatoes
Olives and capers
Small beans such as Mung or Moth
Soy crumbles
Almonds and raisins if you are adventurous

Mix in:
Napa cabbage and Swiss chard chopped
Cilantro chopped
Salt and pepper to taste

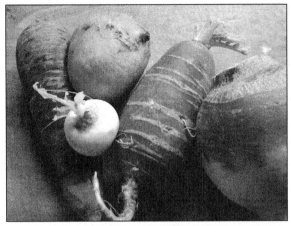

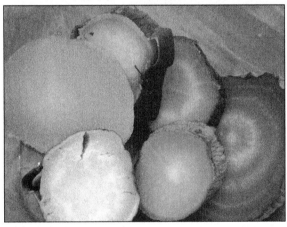

Beets, turnips, and rutabaga, will also cook together. Place in an uncovered baking pan with no water, oil, or condiments, and bake at 400° for an hour. Slices of this delicious and colorful array can complement many a dish. A few years ago I used this photo of the cooked sliced grouping for holiday cards.

BAKED ROOTS, SQUASHES, AND PUMPKINS

Sweet potatoes, potatoes, turnips, and beets can be baked whole without peeling. Squashes such as butternut or acorn and pumpkin like kabocha can be baked whole and in their skin. Place them together in a plain oven proof pan with no grease or water. Bake uncovered at 400° for one hour. At this temperature the natural sugars will caramelize without burning to a bitter taste. Slice to accompany any dish. They refrigerate well for 4-5 days.

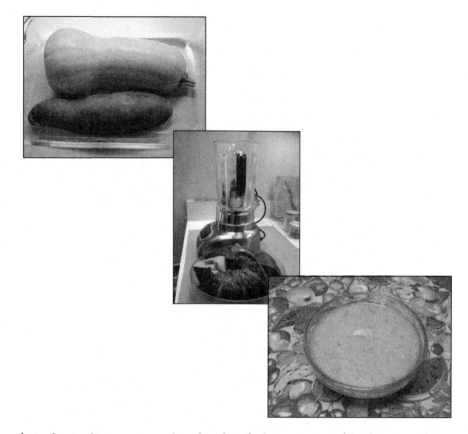

A similar size butternut squash and a white flesh sweet potato (also known as Asian, Korean, or camote in Latin America) bake in the same amount of time—for one hour at 400°.

PUMPKIN AND SWEET POTATO SOUP WITH CASHEWS

Dice a baked sweet potato and twice as much baked squash or pumpkin into the blender.

Add 1/4 cup of raw cashews and enough water for the ingredients to move freely as they grate and blend.

Add a little unsweetened almond milk or light coconut milk for flavor and blend until smooth and creamy.

Add water as you process it until you reach the desired consistency, season with salt and pepper.

Bring out the delicious whole food flavors by heating uncovered before eating.

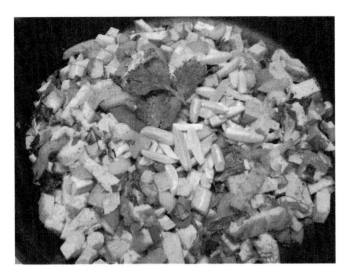

Tofu scramblers owe their appeal to a hearty combination of savory ingredients. The yellow color comes from the similar condiments we use to dye brown or white rice—saffron, turmeric, paprika, and cumin.

TOFU SCRAMBLER

This multicolor dish can include a variety of vegetables and makes a great brunch. The bland tofu block is a good source of vegetable protein and will adapt to your favorite flavors and spices.

1 pound block of extra firm tofu (some brands have substantial amount of calcium, check the nutrition label).
Add turmeric, paprika, saffron, annato, and chipotle. They impart a golden yellow color to the tofu.

1 chopped pepper
1 chopped small onion
1 carrot sliced
1/2 head of broccoli florets
1/2 can diced tomatoes

Discard the tofu water, mash the block, and toss in a hot skillet until most of the water has evaporated leaving it dry and crumbly. Add the yellow powders, reserving the peas and cilantro until the end to keep them from losing their intense green color. Season with salt and pepper. Sprinkle with almonds or chopped walnuts and decorate with sliced olives and capers.

RESOURCES:

1. *Field Guide to Produce, How to Identify, Select, and Prepare Virtually Every Fruit and Vegetable at the Market* by Aliza Green, Quirk Books. A compact easy to use guide with many beautiful color photographs.
2. Food Studies Institute. *Food is Elementary* by Antonia Demas, award winning sensory based nutritional curriculum for children (and curious adults) in place at over three-thousand schools across the country.
3. *Nutrition Guide for Clinicians* published by Physicians Committee for Responsible Medicine.
4. Physicians Committee for Responsible Medicine (PCRM). A national non profit organization which promotes preventive medicine, encourages higher standards in research, and conducts relevant up to date clinical research.
5. *Plant Powered Diet, The Life Long Lasting Plan for Achieving Optimal Health Beginning Today* by Sharon Palmer RD, 2012, The Experiment. This is an excellent encyclopedia of accurate, clear, and concise terms with many recipes. As a person replaces drugs with nourishing foods this book will prove invaluable— a great complement to the one you hold in your hands. Keep a book such as this one on the kitchen counter and refer to it often. Join your child in being curious about the food we eat.
6. Rodale Institute. A nonprofit dedicated to pioneering organic farming through research and outreach. Address: 611 Siegfriedale Rd, Kutztown, PA 19530 (610) 683-6009.
7. *Wellness Foods A to Z* by Sheldon Margen, Edited by University of California at Berkeley. This well organized encyclopedia has color photographs illustrating almost each of the hundreds of foods discussed in alphabetical order, including hints on when and how to buy produce and serving suggestions. Each food is presented with a nutritional breakdown label not required of whole foods in the supermarket but helpful for advancing your food literacy. For example you might be anxious about giving up milk since it is so high in calcium (8 ounces of cow's milk has around 300 milligrams of calcium), until you flip to the page with cooking greens and see that 2 cooked cups of collards have 450 milligrams of calcium!

Part VII

Lessons From Case Studies

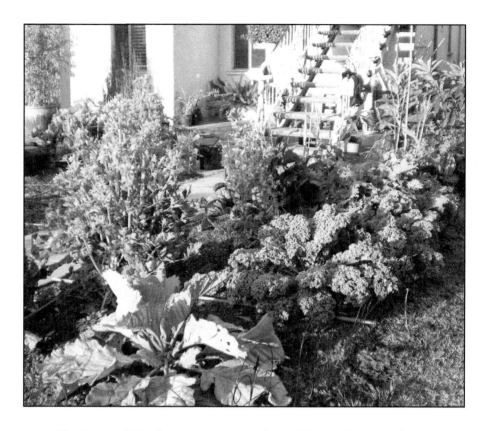

Tend to an edible plant in your surroundings. Observe how, just like us,
it is affected by nourishment and the environment.

Lessons From Case Studies

$\mathcal{M}$y mission with this book has been to reveal some of the body's inner workings and its intimate relationship with food—which is its only source of nourishment. I tried to remove obstacles, such as lack of familiarity with foods or a cluttered kitchen environment. I have aimed to destroy myths and misunderstandings regarding nutrition as well as the cost, time, and effort needed to nourish oneself. My hope is to keep reminding us that the amazing bodies we inhabit are willing to go the distance.

There are as many stories as there are people on what moves one to quit smoking, stay sober, or eat better. It is not always apparent, but some people suddenly feel energized to change when they fall in love, be it with a person, an animal, a project, or the world. At the same time there is little anyone can do to force change on another even though to witness a loved one's persistent unhealthy destructive patterns can be painful. If you feel moved to care for yourself, show gratitude by staying focused.

What follows are excerpts out of the lives of real people. Those who transitioned to a plant based diet felt the benefits within a few weeks. That being the case I would like to report that most made changes for life; that once able to give up medications people didn't gain them back; that those who successfully lost weight did it for good; that those who reduced inflammation chose a future with less pain, more elastic joints, no bloating, and more energy; that those who had a brush with cancer have gone on to support their wellness; that recovering sexual function was enduring motivation, that after the first heart attack people stayed committed to avoid a second one. However, for most the wellness journey is not linear, success happens in fits, spurts, and stages. So with patience, I encourage you to stay the course.

Here are teachings from those who came before you and who show me what I know to be true and how to protect life.

Case Story #1

At only fifty years old, AC was weighing more than eighty pounds her best and hurting. She suffered from high blood pressure and high cholesterol. She had both knees replaced due to painful wear and tear and the gall bladder removed for stones. Diabetic for almost ten years recently had insulin added to her long list of medicines. Over time, AC had followed many diets and had participated in a number of weight loss programs. When she dropped some weight she felt better, but always gained it back. At our first visit AC appeared motivated and agreed to begin a low fat plant based diet. Six weeks later she was amazed. I am full of energy and walking with no pains, it's only been a month and I am off insulin! For six months she was off all medications, but cyclic sets-back tended to catch her by surprise. Losing touch with her core, appointments became sparse, and in a few months she gained back her weight and her medications slipping once again into the frustration and depression that had plagued her since adolescence. Months later AC returned. Motivated by things she wanted to enjoy, this time she focused on her body as a loyal companion deserving utmost care. She kept a very simple monthly plan detailing when she would shop, cook, and freeze and checked it every night before bed. In two months, she felt energy coming from a deep place and was able to stop using insulin again. This time is has been over two years. The goal is to weather future cycles without being thrown completely off balance. She knows she can do it.

Case Study #2

BD came with a BMI of 43 after gaining 150 pounds in three years. At only 27 years old she suffered with constipation, pain in her knees, felt emotionally down, had no energy, and showed little enthusiasm for the successful business she commanded. She gave care and shelter to a dozen abandoned cats, she felt unattractive and bloated. BD was concerned about recent facial hair and wondered if her skin, which had stretched leaving pink lines all over her body, was still elastic. Her young body was breaking down and she couldn't bear it. Never having cooked at home, before our visit she bought a juicer and with head high announced that she was eager to start anew. BD took to our plan the same way she had forged her business with discipline and mastery. Her new foods made into simple recipes became a uniform that she wore every day. Within seven weeks she lost 40 pounds, was spending thirty dollars a week on food instead of thirty dollars a day on take out, and with a big smile she announced: my skin feels clean, my bowels move without effort, the pink lines on my arms and belly are fading, and I have more energy than all my workers combined. I feel beautiful. During that summer BD went with friends on a short beach vacation and ate burgers, French fries, and sweets, for old times sake. She quickly gained five pounds and experienced a negative change in her skin and libido. What a valuable lesson: her body responded to food. BD quickly returned to her "diet" and did it with glee. Last I heard from BD, she had consciously maintained her course and was planning to have liposuction to help her along.

Case Study #3

CE is a faith based vegetarian who has been one-hundred pounds overweight for 30 years. Recently her organism began sending distress signals. Her lipids doubled, her blood pressure was high, her sugars would not come down without insulin, and her knees no longer sustained her without complaint. She came in resenting her medications and the daily blood checks. Shopping and cooking were already part of her routine, so after a short course on food literacy and a few recipes CE said she knew what to do. Within a month she lost ten pounds. She tasted success as sugars normalized and began cutting back on her insulin. In her head she knew what to do, but a long history of impulsive gratification soon looped CE into eating poorly. A nagging internal voice urging her to sabotage her efforts found concrete form in family and friends. Her initial flurry of energy lasted only few months and sadly so did her improvement. She returned feeling achy, weighted down and with high sugars. Sinking into profound sadness she reflects on the gamble she is taking with her future. She walks to the edge of her precipice again and again trying to understand this hunger and it is not for food. CE's difficult task, of letting go her old ways for new life to emerge, is easier said than done. She is teased by friends for declining dinner invitations, still mocked for rejecting cake and ice cream, feels the temptation, and has to constantly renegotiate with people she has shared drink and sweets for many years. Over the past couple of years she has retained some good habits, such as shopping once a week and cooking and freezing meals on a designated day. Much work still lies ahead.

Case Study #4

DF is 63 years old recently divorced lawyer who for the past twenty years has carried 30 extra pounds mostly in a belly that starts below his sternum and looms over his belt. Most of his adult life he has been treated for high blood pressure which he blames on his genes. He also has family history of diabetes, heart disease, and cancer. Recently at the insistence of friends he went to see his doctor for mild persistent discomfort in his chest. Diagnosed with narrowing of his coronary arteries he had a stent put in to improve heart circulation. During our only visit he expressed an intellectual interest in the relationship between diet and heart disease, but would not commit to any significant change. Socially he hangs out with friends who indulge in comfort food and seek out positive reviews for fish, eggs, chicken and olive oil. Like so many of us, he wants to hear good news about his current habits. Waking up is hard to do. I worry for him.

Case Study #5

EJ is a 55 years old executive whose abdomen over the past twenty years had ballooned like a drum. Four months before his visit he was shocked by what he called a small heart attack. He heard about president Bill Clinton's heart doctor from Cleveland Clinic, Caldwell Esselstyn, and subscribed to his plan. Being a good cook, he started a low fat plant based diet and within little more than a month he had lost 20 pounds energetically announcing plans to arrest and reverse his heart disease. Unfortunately, his urgency dissipated before achieving target weight and he drifted back to a diet of moderation, yet as Doctor Esselstyn says moderation kills. It was only a short time before he gained back most of the weight and therefore his risks. At his job he is expected to sing the merits of milk, cheese, and yogurt, foods which he had initially cut out as part of his personal recovery. It is not easy to serve these two masters.

Case Study #6

FH used to play sports in college, but not being in organized sports anymore, he grew a bit heavier each year. Then he got married and became a Dad. Today he is 30 years old, ninety pounds overweight, and on regular medicine for acid reflux. FH remembers being raised on pasta, meats, pizza, deli sandwiches, chips, yogurt, milk, and string cheese. Last year, the family went on a week long vacation where unbeknownst to them were served only low fat plant fare. He was amazed that even though he piled up food on his plate as usual, he did not feel bloated. Within three days he confessed to his spouse that he did not need his acid pill. A week later they all returned home to the usual food and children to a school that fails to come to their rescue. His obese partner, a vegetarian but not a plant eater, feeds the family mostly heavy processed foods and cheese, with token amounts of broccoli, spinach, bananas, and baby carrots. The short week free of symptoms and medicines now remains tucked in an album of fading memories. Absent a kitchen laboratory where they would learn food literacy and the value of cooking whole foods, the children are likely follow in their parents' footsteps, or perhaps not.

Case Study #7

GI is 33 and although he grew up eating rice, beans, kale, collards, and sweet potatoes, when he came to the U.S. he fell in love with all you can eat buffets, fried chicken, soda, and our daily bread. In three years he gained 80 pounds and a sundry of symptoms, which made him seek medical attention. A persistent cough and constant fatigue were diagnosed as gastro-esophageal reflux and sleep apnea. Blood pressure and triglycerides were off the charts. He suffered clinical depression, which left him unmotivated and feeling lousy. He accepted a CPAP machine for his sleep apnea (to get enough oxygen at night) and resigned himself to several pills a day for everything else. Visits to doctors became more frequent than visits to the barber. He was irritable all the time and always out of breath and shortly began using an asthma inhaler—his work and his family suffered. Then one morning something snapped. He woke up not wanting to hurt anyone by being sick all the time. A surge of what he called self respect welled up inside of him. He started eating less, began cooking his greens, going to the gym six days a week, and consciously eliminating negative words. There was nothing manic about his behavior. It was a deliberate change of course. He lost the 80 pounds he had gained, unplugged his apnea machine, and no longer needed medications for anything. He felt content and capable of caring for himself. Three years later remains relentlessly committed and believes love moved him to do what fear never did. His wife, on the other hand, won't jostle their two kids, appeasing them with candy, bread, fast food, cheese, soda, cake, and ice cream. For the past two years they have received warning letters from school regarding the youngest child's increasing BMI. Schools can and must do so much more than send letters home.

Case Study #8

At only 42 HJ has a long history of antacid use for digestive complaints. Multiple endoscopies always show gastritis. Repeat treatments grant her only temporary relief. Her excess twenty pounds are mostly due to bread, chicken, milk and juice. She eats very few vegetables or fruits. Committed to everyone but herself she insists that changing the way she cooks would be unfair to her demanding family. She was absent from care for many months and when she returned it was with persistent pains after gall bladder surgery. This time her triglycerides were 600 (normal for this blood lipid is 100). Impressed by my urgency she agreed to a drastic change of diet that would consist on eliminating meats and dairy and eat mostly produce. In one week and without medications her triglycerides came down to 175 and her pain was almost gone. For the first time she had palpable evidence of what her diet could accomplish, yet caring for herself remains buried under the many obligations she feels for others. How might she help her family eat healthier when messages from her own body come through lines of communication that are frail and noisy with static?

Case Study #9

I saw AB for the first time when he was 5 years old, short for his age, pale, and thin. He walked in accompanied by his anguished mom, dad, and older sister. They confessed living in constant fear of AB's next asthma attack and the dreaded emergency room visits. The parents diligently administered the inhaler treatments and everyone constantly reminded him not to run or exert himself. His school attendance was spotty in spite of compliance with the current treatment. He looked at me with big eyes as I listened to the whistles and wheezes coming out of his chest. A review of his diet uncovered that he ate a pound of string cheese a week, all by himself. Some people produce a disproportionate amount of leukotrienes from the arachidonic acid in dairy and meat. Leukotrienes are potent broncho-constrictors. We discussed this and the parents were so hopeful that they agreed to gladly eliminate cheese not just for him, but for the entire household. A month later I saw AB and his family again. This time they were smiling. AB's weight was catching up, his demeanor was curious, outgoing, and he beamed. As I listened with my stethoscope, he smiled pointing to the center of his chest and said I don't hurt here anymore. AB didn't know his chest hurt until it did not! Many adult people walk into a jail of symptoms and discomforts without realizing they can walk out, the cell door is wide open.

Case Study #10

For many years mom catered to dad's limited taste. As a result she too ate very poorly. At 86, her small frame was thirty pounds overweight, she felt fatigued, suffered with severe joint pains, had high blood pressure, and seemed unsteady in her feet. She felt achy all the time, could not make a fist, and slept very poorly. She began using a cane and was told she needed new knees. Then my father died. Very sad and without a firm grasp of her functional capacity I invited her to come stay with me for a couple of weeks. From the moment she stepped in the house she had no meat, cheese, or refined foods; she ate only plants and lots of them. I watched her during the day recover lost sleep during long and frequent naps. After ten days of eating an abundance of plants, especially cruciferous, and walking up and down the house stairs, she announced she wanted to cook with me. She could make a tight fist, felt elastic, and marveled that she was sleeping through the night. That initial visit extended to a whole month, during which we walked uneven terrain, hiked blooming gardens, and even paddled a canoe. She shed most of her extra weight and dropped ten inches from her waist enabling her to bend and tie her shoes. She forgot to use her cane around the house. Physically and emotionally she was gaining life back. She said her only regret was not starting sooner! Our long visits turned regular. Her whole plant menu grew and we laughed on the phone as she confessed she was adding more vegetables than the recipes called for. Three years later as she celebrated her eighty-ninth birthday, she was still cooking favorite and new dishes every day; proudly lecturing to family, friends, plumbers, and priests, on everything she knew first hand about the diet that restored her wellbeing. Of course it was more than diet, it must have included a spark of life from within and invisible to the outside eye. Find yours.

Case Study #11

CD found out he was diabetic about eight years ago, he is now in his early 40s. His wife is also diabetic as well as her whole family. Relatives of the couple on both sides have succumbed to diabetic complications including amputations and early deaths. Their two adolescent children, already obese, are following in their footsteps. CD comes in for care very sporadically seeing different physicians each time who keep adding more medications in an attempt to bring his blood sugars within range. During the office visits the couple listens to food and diabetes education and agree to half baked plans, but remain frustratingly defiant eating fried foods, sweets, meat, cheese, and bread, on a daily basis. Neither he nor his wife have been able to make salutary changes. They regard cooking once a week and packing a daily lunch as nearly impossible. I was surprised one morning when he appeared wanting to reconnect. On three medications, his blood sugar was almost five hundred (normal being in the range of 70 to 120). As usual he reported not making any changes in his eating habits and admitted indulging regularly at the end of the day and on weekends for stress release. The presence of ketones in his urine told me his body was burning fat for energy instead of glucose and with triple his previous average sugars I persuaded him to start insulin. He acted very surprised. I listened to his objections on how impossible it would be to check sugars and use insulin given his work schedule, but welling up with tears he agreed. Since the weekend was approaching, I would call him the next few mornings to check on his progress. Besides starting insulin, he needed to improve sensitivity to insulin by eliminating meats, cheese, and other saturated fats, plus he needed to eat close to a pound of plants, especially cruciferous, every day. He left with a short shopping list and a couple of recipes—promising to do his best. The first night he reported waking up with a sensation of blood rushing into his legs. The next two mornings, he couldn't believe it when he woke up with an erection, an event he hadn't experienced for two years. His sugars were still in the 200 range, but arterial elasticity had improved almost immediately (thanks to endothelial nitric oxide). This delightful couple does justice to the refrain that it takes two to tango. She remains restless, unyielding, rebellious even, not wanting to lose her childish innocence. AG continues to live his routine in automatic pilot until the morning of his next appointment when his stress level rises in the face of his own betrayal, but has become less scared and more independent showing better understanding of his inner body workings. There is hope.

Case Study #12

EF, EI, EO are some of the many people who live with chronic back pain attributed to various causes, from arthritis to fibromyalgia to spinal stenosis. They came following a long list of treatment failures including analgesics, antidepressants, opiods, and nerve anesthetizing drugs injected into the spinal canal. For each of them pain, the crude language with which the body expresses distress, figured in daily activities, work, sleep, and anything else that had to be planned with omnipresent feelings of frustration, depression, and hopelessness.

At our initial visit we took a Virtual Tour of their respective Kitchens. On the counters were cereal boxes, bread, and bananas. In the fridge were spinach, zucchini, string beans, apples, grapes, celery, and cole slaw mix, with 1% and 2% milk, ice tea, juices, eggs, butter, lunch meats, left over Chinese, cheeses, and yogurt. In the freezer were chicken, hot dogs, lean cuisines, turkey burgers, rye bread, beef stew, chicken breasts, pork chops, hot sausages, fish sticks, peas, fresh fruit popsicles, bagels, waffles, and French toast. The cupboards were stocked with peanut butter and jelly, pasta, canned vegetables, rice, canned beans, instant oats, cookies, chips, nutty bars, microwave popping corn, almonds, spray oil, olive oil, and canola oil. Two had recently eliminated regular soda and other sweet drinks from the house. We agreed that the balance of foods favored animal and processed items which from a nutritional stand point are associated with inflammation. The sparse presence of antioxidant rich plant foods in their food banks paled against the preponderance of calories from saturated fat, sugars, flour, and animal protein. Since these foods produce inflammation which fuels pain, we planned a transition to a plant based kitchen. (Refer to the first chapter of this book) Each took to this plan at least in the short term. Each was surprised with their bodies' fast response regarding less pain to more elasticity, increased energy, and a sharper mind. Besides improved back pain, one patient had no more migraines, another stopped the pain medicines he had been on for years, and yet another cancelled her next epidural injection intended to numb her back nerves! What will each do with this living experience? How will they support this new possibility? If we had gravel inside our shoes we wouldn't think of numbing our feet so they would not feel pain, we would clean out our shoes of the culprit pebbles.

Case Study #13

GH is 28 years old and has never been to doctors for anything serious. Today he brought his mother for follow up of gall bladder surgery. Since he seemed about fifteen pounds over weight and his diet consisted of takeout and fast food on the job, I offered to check his lipids. His triglycerides were over 600 (normal for this blood fat is less than 100). His mood turned serious and we spent half hour going over the foods he would eliminate, foods that would take their place, templates for basic recipes, and portion size. His homework was to stop drinking beer, to cook and pack a lunch. I would see him back in one week. A week later triglycerides had dropped to 230 without medications putting a smile of relief and accomplishment on his face. He was eating oats in the morning, cooking greens during the week, and packing a lunch for work every day. Eating like this was not hard. Fending off jabs from pizza eating coworkers who accused him of being extreme was far more difficult. After two weeks GH's triglycerides were 110, he had dropped eight pounds, felt energetic, and had returned to the soccer field. He remained confused by comments from family and friends who wondered whether he was losing weight because he was sick. With continuing education and support GH developed more confidence. Soon he had strong arguments in defense of his new lifestyle. At six month follow up, GH had begun to test the boundaries of his food choices bringing triglycerides up to the 300 range. This time he knew exactly why and instead of responding with gloom he met the news with renewed determination. He now looks his age with a trim and fit body of which he is proud and most importantly he is much more aware of how he can protect his health.

Case Study #14

When IJ walked in to see me, every step was punctuated by a pained expression on her face. She had been diagnosed with rheumatoid arthritis based on clinical and laboratory tests and had been on two drugs including methotrexate, a common rheumatoid arthritis medication. On moderate dose prednisone (a strong anti inflammatory drug) she still hurt and if she ran out the swelling and joint pains came back with a vengeance. She consumed very few vegetables, ate mostly processed foods, meats, cheese, fruits and fruit juices. We spent some time discussing inflammation and food literacy then came up with a plan for her. She would eliminate dairy products and fruit juices, cut out all red meat and as most chicken as she could. She would nourish herself with cruciferous vegetables, legumes, oats, fruits, and a few nuts. We anticipated cutting back her moderate dose prednisone in a few weeks. She was about fifteen pounds overweight, which contributed to her inflammation, but we would not focus on this initially. Immediately as she began her new eating plan her hands and feet stopped hurting and joint swelling went down. She walked up to her next appointment with a smile, had lost about 8 pounds, and contemplated getting back to work. She was slowly weaned off her prednisone and finally discontinued it with no recurring pain or swelling. She made durable changes in her diet and how well she feels continues to be her motivation. It has been almost four years.

Case Study #15 Mom, Dad, Two girls, One boy

I met Mom almost twenty years ago. As she formed a family I had the privilege of greeting its new members. When those living abroad came to visit, one of their first stops was to meet me. During the twelve years I have cooked with my patients, the youngest was born and the other celebrated her sweet sixteen.

Mom shares the head of the household with a kind large man who provides for the family and whose only medical problem is high blood lipids. The family's changes in eating have been not as impressive as their enormous growth in plant food literacy. This year, the oldest girl announced to the family that she is following a plant diet. Mom felt her own support would be inadequate and came to me. Over the years I have given away copies of a book to such teens, titled *A Teen's Guide to Going Vegetarian* by Judy Krizmanic (published by Puffin in 1994). I was able to pull out one of these treasures for Mom and her daughter, who will translate its pages for the family—the ripples of cognizance run in all directions.

Case Study #16

UV's restaurant was selected to cater a local health event for which I too was consulted. Our discussions over the event menu brought up her own discomfort with excess weight, acid reflux, and migraine. UV was a quick study. A few weeks later her restaurant delivered a tasty low fat plant based spread which had everyone raving enthusiastically. After a short follow up and an informal personal session she decided to go plant based for a while. To her surprise she did not have another migraine, was off reflux medicine almost immediately, and in two weeks had lost 7 pounds which she announced with an incredulous smile. A very touching report came from her sweetheart who happily has not heard her snore again. As her life becomes come congruent, she projects that the restaurant will undergo changes reflecting her own.

Case Study #17

WX was diabetic during her last pregnancy. Her sugars came down after giving birth, but she remained very overweight and followed no specific nutritional plan. Five years later she came with daily headaches, feeling fatigued, and clueless as to the cause. Her blood sugar was over 300. A virtual tour of her kitchen revealed mostly chicken, juice, bread, milk, and boxed cereals. She snacked at work on fruit, deli meats, cheese, and pretzels. After a short session she agreed to discover for herself what would happen if she eliminated meats and dairy and ate only plant foods for a few weeks. She left on no medications. Two days later her sugar was 106, she had no more headaches and felt energized. The challenge now, as with most people in her predicament, is to maintain this new lifestyle and return to her normal weight, so that diabetes does not become her default health status.

Case Study #18

AE worked as a cook in a restaurant when one day was taken to the local emergency room with dizziness and chest pain. Having no symptoms and being only 51 years old, he had chosen to ignore his high blood pressure. This time it was so high it was causing his heart to beat very fast and very irregular. After two days in the hospital he was released on blood pressure medications for out patient follow up. On the day we met we discussed the blood viscosity and inflammation associated with his meat diet. He carried 15 extra pounds mostly around his waist and although his lipids were within normal range, dropping this weight would help normalize blood pressure. With the scary event still fresh in his memory AE took to a mostly plant diet, dropped 8 pounds, and his blood pressure remained normal on half the original dose of medications. Months went by and his appointments began to lapse, his medication refills were spotty, and when I saw him again, he had an asymptomatic blood pressure of 180/120 (normal should top at 140/80). I told him half in jest that this time it was I the one about to have a heart attack. His wife works longer hours, so he does most of the food shopping and cooking. She is 35 pounds above the weight she carried at age twenty, so it would benefit both to agree on a nourishment plan. Since she was in the waiting room, with his permission we invited her in. The conversation that ensued included a brief exposé of high blood pressure risks then moved on to a virtual tour of their kitchen, a list of food preferences, an assessment of their cooking competence, and concluded with a cursory food budget emphasizing fresh plants plus three recipes they could prepare with the foods they had in the kitchen on that same day. Adding only half a pill of a medication he had taken in the past, AE agreed to eliminate meats and processed foods and return for a blood pressure check in one week. He came back as planned this time sporting a blood pressure of 140/80. Reporting he had not cheated in a week he gave me the most heartfelt bear hug of my life. When we are in each others lives with love and care and support, we have the time of our lives. This couple has found a way to renew their commitment to a healthy life together and are giving an enduring example to their adolescent daughter.

Case Study #19

CW is a construction worker. Our visit started with his desire to get cholesterol under control. Like many people of his generation, he grew up on home cooked meals, but today he is away from family and works around younger people who survive on pizza and take-out, watch TV, and drink beer to unwind. After a short chat he offered the following insight—I have been taking the path of least resistance. High ground can be lonely, so one tends to ignore the stirrings of discomfort—he went on exploring what all this meant for his life today and I watched him recover sit straighter and smile. Inside his brawny exterior is a sensitive man who respects his body and is moved by beauty in nature. He left determined to seek members of his tribe—by this he meant spend time in the company of people who share his sense of purpose. Three months later his lipids were only slightly lower but he had found delight in cooking and more compatible company for leisure activities. Someone once said, be the change you want to see in the world.

Case Study #20

YZ came carrying her sturdy 5' 6" frame and 210 pounds with aching elegance. She was suffering with painful joints, frequent headaches, and consti-pation. Her daily nutrition consisted of meats, cheese, some fruits, and bread. She liked vegetables but ate them sparingly as side dish. Her laboratory studies showed no outstanding abnormalities in lipids, sugars, or arthritis markers, but she was not well. Her social and religious life includes doing most of the cooking for communal eating. Giving up food items her friends expect at the table was not an option for YZ. However she was able to eliminate milk, cheese, most meats, and began to eat leafy greens every day. In spite of only a modest weight loss of ten pounds, she had almost immediate resolution of her pains and a return to normal bowel function. With a big smile head high and swinging arms YZ remarks that she's done good.

Case Study #21

For four or five years, CZ dealt very tangentially with his diagnosis of diabetes. Blame was not in short supply as he refused to take control of his diet and placed the responsibility on his wife. The marriage was stable but unsatisfactory and one day it dissolved. When I began to see CZ again, he had regrouped entering in a mutually supportive relationship. However, this time he did not hand his health over to his partner, instead he charted a plan for success which was solidly his. In the course of a year, blood sugars dropped and remained normal, Hemoglobin A1c (which averages the blood sugars of the previous three months) went from 11 to 7 (normal), blood lipids dropped and remained normal, blood pressure remains normal. Today he is on no medication.

Case Study #22

FM had lost seven pounds in a month. Under better circumstances this would have been good news, but she felt fatigued and thirsty. Her blood sugar in the office was 496 and the hemoglobin A1c >14 indicating that average blood sugars in the past three months were over 300. Unbeknownst to her she had become diabetic. With her four year old at her side, FM digested the news and accepted the plan to eliminate meat, cheese, processed foods, and sugary drinks which she was using to quench her thirst and to rehydrate with water and slowly increase plant foods. Family support was essential so she could rest and care for herself. She started metformin to temporarily improve insulin sensitivity, learned to check her sugars, and we brushed up on some simple recipes—all this without the benefit of reading or writing skills. FM made substantial changes in her life with the precious support of her husband and in two months her blood sugars consistently in the 90s we discontinued her medication. In one more month her hemoglobin A1c had dropped to 6.9. Today she beams with joy feeling empowered to protect her health and that of her family.

Last thought for now: Embody the change you want.

Epilogue

*W*e owe praise to the ethical relationships that between pharmaceutical industry and physicians have unquestionably improved our lives. However, much has been written about the imprint, in great measure unconscious, of a pharmaceutical industry whose insidious presence in the medical setting affects not only our prescribing, but our attitude toward a health care system over-reliant on drugs.

As young doctors in the hospital, whenever we needed respite we would go to the residents lounge. I hardly ever saw a faculty member enter this refuge and yet I remember that the "drug reps" as we called them came in freely always bearing gifts of pizza and soda or doughnuts and coffee. I remember they were friendly, young like us, and wore suits. Some sat to defend their drugs to anyone who would listen, those more tactful waited to catch us in the more professional atmosphere of the clinic where they showed up with pens, note pads, and magnets.

I was aware throughout my training of futile attempts by faculty, nurses, and receptionists to rein in their presence, for example at one point the drug reps were required to make an appointment to meet with the doctor rather than drop in with samples expecting a few minutes of our time. I was slippery and avoided being scheduled. Occasionally I was cornered to sign for drug samples, but I refused to be captive audience to their spiels. I felt that listening to their ads would unavoidably influence me. When instead of their gift books (advertisement for their drug) I requested text books, they seldom arrived. I felt that if the manufacturing company paid for its own research the new drug's reported benefits could be biased, so I created a boundary for myself.

We practiced medicine surrounded with mugs and trinkets emblazoned with trade mark drug names. Every surface, shelf, and drawer colonized by ads. Like seeds stuck to the soles of our shoes, these items traveled with us far and wide. Somehow I ended up with a red two inch Swiss army knife. I like the damn gadget which still reads: Ten-K potassium chloride—The Versatile K. The hospital offered drug sponsored conferences and if not lured by the topic people would come in for the food. When I overheard colleagues accepting tickets to sport or orchestra events, I felt embarrassed for them and kept these offers at bay. I did not attend drug sponsored conferences held at fancy restaurants and at medical conventions I did not pick up their tote bags, kitchen spatulas, or flip flops.

It took active decision on my part as a young physician to not go with the flow. I subscribed to The Lancet, a medical journal free of advertisements. During the early years I stayed abreast of new and reviewed drugs reading The Medical Letter and later relied on Prescriber's Letter, neither accept drug sponsors. Today I resonate with the expressed values of PharmedOut founded by Adrianne Fugh-Berman, MD, in 2006, "a Georgetown University Medical Center project that advances evidence-based prescribing and educates healthcare professionals about pharmaceutical marketing practices."

Glossary

Antioxidants: are molecules that can safely interact with free radicals and stop damage from being inflicted on our vital molecules. Some of the most potent antioxidants are found in plants.

Calories represent units of energy.

Condiment: anything added to a dish—such as lemon or vinegar, herbs and ground seeds, or small amounts of strong ingredients such as garlic, ginger, olives, or fennel—to enhance flavor.

Food literacy: the educated state of recognizing whole and processed foods, making sense of nutrition labels, generally knowing how to cook, and having a broad understanding of how the body uses food for nourishment.

Free radicals: unstable atoms or groups of atoms which form when oxygen interacts with certain molecules. Highly unstable, due to its unpaired number of electrons, a free radical stabilizes by reacting with any other molecule that can lend it an electron. When free radicals react with our DNA (genetic material) or the cell membrane, they can cause vital cells to function poorly or die.

Grams and milligrams represent weight (mass).

Macrophages: important cells part of our immune system. Macrophages are large cells strategically located throughout the body and charged with eating, processing, and eliminating foreign materials, dead cells and debris. They recruit additional macrophages in response to inflammatory signals.

Oil: highly refined product overused in cooking. Oil is 100 calories per tablespoon, 100% fat.

Ounces: sometimes refer to dry weight and at other times represent fluid volume.

Paradox: a statement that seems self contradictory.

Phytochemicals: substances naturally occurring in plants.

Plant Based diet: composed mostly of unrefined plants (raw and cooked) with only small amounts of factory processed foods.

Plant based milks: liquid squeezed out of grains, nuts, or seeds, which have been ground and soaked in water. Common plant based milks include soymilk, almond milk, rice milk, hemp, and coconut milk. They are often supplemented with calcium to help some people who do not consume enough vegetables meet the dietary requirements of this mineral. Watch out for those with added sugars.

Refined: factory processed ingredients that no longer resemble the mother food from where they were extracted. For example sugar, oil, and flour. Refined foods are not found in nature. Naturally occurring concentrations of minerals (salts) are found in dunes and flats—however, plants take minerals from the soil and store them in roots, leaves, fruits, and seeds, from where we can access them in proportional amounts.

Sugar: a highly refined product overused in processed foods. Sugar in all its permutations is 60 calories per tablespoon and 100% carbohydrate with none of the benefits of its plant of origin.

Titanic: a British passenger liner that sank in 1912 after colliding with an iceberg. The common expression rearranging the deck chairs on the Titanic refers to making cosmetic changes while refusing to change course that could avert disaster.

Vegan: one who does not use or consume any animal products.

Vitamins: compounds necessary for the normal function of our bodies and which we need in very small amounts. The body can make Vitamin A (from carotenes), Vitamin D (on skin exposed to sunlight) and Vitamin K (through bacteria in our gut). All other vitamins (B group, C, and E) are found in plant foods. Although bacteria make Vitamin B_{12} in our colon, we absorb it proximally in the small intestine, so we all need this supplement.

Volume is measured in gallons, cups, liters, milliliters, tablespoons, and teaspoons.

Whole foods: are easily recognized because they are as they appear in nature. Except for grains, nuts, and seeds, which need to be collected and bagged for market, whole foods have not been altered. They come to us as that part of the plant that we most likely use for food—root, leaves, stem, crown, or fruit.

Zonulin: a protein that modulates the permeability of tight junctions between cells of the wall of the digestive tract.

Acknowledgements

*M*any people have mentored me—their teachings are woven into my life, however those I mention here gave more than a spark to this project. My mom, Trina Gelabert, loving, wise, and lifelong fan—she lived nourishing the body and recovering health to her very end. My son, Jason Binnick, a sharp and warm accomplished composer, always in my corner mirroring loving compassion, discipline, and confidence. John Robbins, my hero, split open the hearts of scientists like myself with *Diet For A New America* and our world was never the same. Antonia Demas, of Food Studies Institute, friend and mentor—with her I took my first steps in rigorous plant food education. Jim Gordon and Susan B. Lord of The Center for Mind Body Medicine, helped me and many physicians advance our medical nutrition education when no one else was doing it. Neal Barnard, of Physicians Committee for Responsible Medicine—a torchbearer, clear of mind, and unwavering supporter. And all those whose commitment to more responsible medicine preceded mine—leaving mileposts along the way—I hold each one dear.

Whenever I was encouraged to write a book, I would reply that I was living it. Then I felt the stirrings of new life and my son designed me a website—a gift I still cherish. Today the body of my work is in these pages where a few of you have left fingerprints and scratch marks as it progressed through various stages: Janet Baldo, Idalia Capó, Marilyn Furfari, Bonita Janzen, Paulette Kouffman, Tina Smith.

I am grateful to those who ventured outside of their field to comment on the book—John Robbins, Jonathan Balcombe, Howard Jacobson, Sharon Palmer, Susan Silberstein, Koshy Mathews, Jeffrey I. Mechanick, Tom Tobin, Fred de Long, Sharon Wylie, Barry Jacobs, Jeffrey Mechanick, Vance Lehmkuhl, Antonia Demas, Vera Andrus, Anthony Sparano, Eileen Bowe. Heartfelt thanks go to Jane Heil, who expertly guided the task of putting together manuscript submissions.

I am inspired by those who come to me as patients—you continue to demonstrate the undeniable connection between nourishment and health.

Finally I am indebted to my publisher at Sunstone Press, James Clois Smith, Jr., who handled this project with the respect and expertise that I wish every author could get. Thank you.

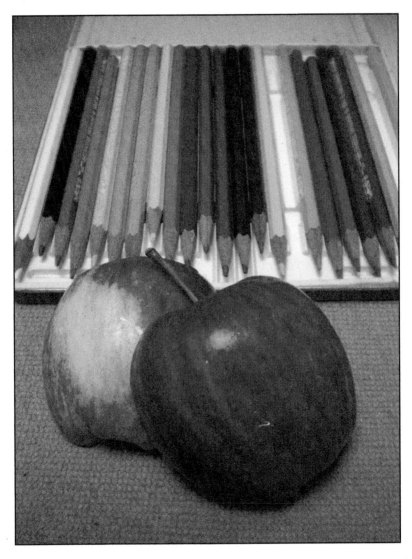

Nature concentrates nutrients of various aromas, flavors, and textures, exclusively in plants enticing all living animals including humans, with the colors of the rainbow.

Index

CPSIA information can be obtained
at www.ICGtesting.com
Printed in the USA
BVOW11s0726180516

448544BV00032B/303/P